WRITING
RESEARCH PROPOSALS
IN THE HEALTH SCIENCES

Sara Miller McCune founded SAGE Publishing in 1965 to support the dissemination of usable knowledge and educate a global community. SAGE publishes more than 1000 journals and over 800 new books each year, spanning a wide range of subject areas. Our growing selection of library products includes archives, data, case studies and video. SAGE remains majority owned by our founder and after her lifetime will become owned by a charitable trust that secures the company's continued independence.

Los Angeles | London | New Delhi | Singapore | Washington DC | Melbourne

WRITING
RESEARCH PROPOSALS
IN THE HEALTH SCIENCES
A STEP–BY–STEP GUIDE

ZEVIA SCHNEIDER
& JEFFREY FULLER

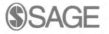

Los Angeles | London | New Delhi
Singapore | Washington DC | Melbourne

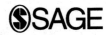

Los Angeles | London | New Delhi
Singapore | Washington DC | Melbourne

SAGE Publications Ltd
1 Oliver's Yard
55 City Road
London EC1Y 1SP

SAGE Publications Inc.
2455 Teller Road
Thousand Oaks, California 91320

SAGE Publications India Pvt Ltd
B 1/I 1 Mohan Cooperative Industrial Area
Mathura Road
New Delhi 110 044

SAGE Publications Asia-Pacific Pte Ltd
3 Church Street
#10-04 Samsung Hub
Singapore 049483

Editor: Becky Taylor
Assistant editor: Charlène Burin
Production editor: Katie Forsythe
Indexer: David Rudeforth
Marketing manager: Tamara Navaratnam
Cover design: Wendy Scott
Typeset by: C&M Digitals (P) Ltd, Chennai, India
Printed in the UK

Library of Congress Control Number: 2017949299

British Library Cataloguing in Publication data

A catalogue record for this book is available from
the British Library

ISBN 978-1-5264-1130-3
ISBN 978-1-5264-1131-0 (pbk)

At SAGE we take sustainability seriously. Most of our products are printed in the UK using FSC papers and boards.
When we print overseas we ensure sustainable papers are used as measured by the PREPS grading system.
We undertake an annual audit to monitor our sustainability.

CONTENTS

ABOUT THE AUTHORS

Zevia Schneider was Associate Professor: Research and Co-ordinator of Higher Degrees by Research in the Faculty of Nursing at the Royal Melbourne Institute of Technology University, and then Director of Post Graduate Studies in the Faculty of Education. She has co-authored five editions of *Nursing and Midwifery Research: methods and appraisal for evidence-based practice*, with the 5th edition published in 2016. She has been involved in a range of funded research projects in the fields of pregnancy, antenatal services, early discharge from hospital, distance education, and programme evaluation.

Zevia has been an invited guest speaker, receiving an invitation from the Ministry of Education in Brunei to conduct a workshop for community health nurses, and has presented papers at national and international conferences. She has completed a PhD in the Faculty of Education at Monash University. Her specialist research area is pregnancy, and in particular the role of the couple as educator of their infant.

Jeffrey Fuller is Emeritus Professor of Nursing at Flinders University with a background in primary health care service quality and safety, integrated care, leadership, health care service evaluation, and research capacity building in qualitative and quantitative methods. He was the Associate Dean (Research) in the Flinders School of Nursing & Midwifery from 2012 to 2015. He has completed 30 research-to-practice projects since 2000 in collaborative models of chronic illness care in Australia and China, and he is the author of a large number of research papers all conducted in partnership with service organizations so as to ensure relevance and implementation. Prior to academia, he was the team leader of a community health service in the northern Adelaide region of South Australia. In 2015, he was awarded the Basil Hetzel Leadership Award in Public Health from the Public Health Association of Australia.

AUTHORS' ACKNOWLEDGEMENTS

We are two academics committed to facilitating skills in the writing of clear and logical research proposals. Our motivation for writing this guide stems from many years of reviewing research proposals for postgraduate studies, research committees, ethics committees, grant funding committees, and through supervision of higher degree students.

Our main audiences for this guide are higher degree students and early career researchers in the health care sciences. Higher degree students are required to complete a research proposal when applying for candidature in a research Masters or PhD. Early career researchers need to write research proposals that are competitive in order to succeed in securing grants.

The production of this guide was facilitated by the SAGE UK publishing team. We would like to express our gratitude and appreciation to Charlène Burin, Assistant Editor, Nursing & Health; Becky Taylor, Publisher, Psychology & Health; Alex Clabburn, Commissioning Editor; Katie Forsythe, Senior Production Editor; and Wendy Scott, Senior Designer at SAGE Publishing, for their cooperation, encouragement and guidance throughout the writing process.

We gratefully acknowledge the copyright holders, Elsevier Australia, Flinders University and the Health Research Board of Ireland, for granting permission to reproduce their works in the guide.

We are indebted to our families and colleagues who patiently and enthusiastically provided advice, encouragement and support. Zevia thanks Mina, Cheryl, Saul, Anne and Brenda. Jeff thanks Leonie. He also thanks Pam Smith, the Flinders University Research Manager with whom he worked for a number of years to develop proposal writing capacity amongst many new researchers.

To the readers of the guide, we hope that you enjoy meeting Natasha and Liang and that their enthusiasm and commitment to the research process will stimulate and encourage you to write your own proposal.

PUBLISHER'S ACKNOWLEDGEMENTS

The publisher would like to thank the following individuals for their invaluable feedback on the proposal of and chapters in the book:

Jennifer Boddy

Carrie Jo Braden

Jaqualyn Moore

Claire Peers

The authors and publisher would also like to thank Niraj Rai and Charlène Burin for their impersonation of Liang and Natasha, as well as the following for their kind permission to reproduce material:

Table 3.1 Comparison of approaches to data analysis of popular qualitative methodologies, Schneider et al., (2016) *Nursing and Midwifery Research: methods and appraisal for evidence-based practice* 5th edn. Australia: Elsevier. Reproduced with permission.

Table 3.2 Continuum of quantitative research designs, Schneider et al., (2016) *Nursing and Midwifery Research: methods and appraisal for evidence-based practice* 5th edn. Australia: Elsevier. Reproduced with permission.

Table 6.1 Categories to assess level of risk (Flinders University of South Australia), Research Services Office at the University of Flinders, Australia. Reproduced with kind permission.

Table 6.2 Main topics covered in an application to the Social and Behavioural Ethics Committee (Flinders University of South Australia), Research Services Office at the University of Flinders, Australia. Reproduced with kind permission.

Table 7.1 Sections in a template for a small grant, drawn from the template of the Faculty of Medicine, Nursing and Health Sciences, Flinders University of South Australia. Reproduced with kind permission.

Appendix A: Critical review guidelines for qualitative studies, Schneider et al., (2016) *Nursing and Midwifery Research: methods and appraisal for evidence-based practice* 5th edn. Australia: Elsevier. Reproduced with permission.

Appendix B: Critical review guidelines for quantitative studies, Schneider et al., (2016) *Nursing and Midwifery Research: methods and appraisal for evidence-based practice* 5th edn. Australia: Elsevier. Reproduced with permission.

Appendix D: Sections in a template for a large grant, Template of the Emerging Investigator Awards of the Health Research Board of Ireland. Reproduced with kind permission.

ABOUT THE BOOK

HOW TO USE THIS STEP-BY-STEP GUIDE

This book is a step-by-step guide to help you to work through the various sections of writing a research proposal, whether this is for a thesis or dissertation review committee, an ethical review committee or a grant funding committee.

The book is divided into seven steps as follows, each representing a stage in the research proposal: from proposal preparation; background and justification for the study; research approach and design; abstract, title and significance; feasibility, track record and teams; ethical and legal issues; and writing a funding proposal. It is laid out in this way because writing a proposal is built up stepwise. Each step contains distinct tasks, from canvassing the early general idea of a research question/problem to the final rigorous and polished proposal. The step-by-step icon is intended to reinforce the idea that writing a proposal is a careful and deliberate process of passing from one step to the next in a particular order.

The following chapters of this guide line up with the sequence of steps to write a research proposal. Table i.1 on the following page shows these steps as well as the considerations and activities involved in developing a research proposal.

As you work through the book you will be introduced to two fictional health science characters, Natasha and Liang. Each has a different research question/problem to which you will be progressively introduced as they develop their research proposals in steps. There will be exercises, related to their proposals, for you to complete. After completing these hypothetical exercises, there will be a section for you to complete about your own research problem and plan. At the end of the guide, you should have completed a research proposal that you can use, with the relevant reformatting, to send to a review committee.

If you are writing a proposal as part of a research higher degree, you may wish to work through this guide with your supervisors.

OUR ASSUMPTION

This guide is not a research text book. To get the most out of the book we have assumed that you have already completed a course on research methods and that you have access to research text books. Depending upon your place of work, you will also have the occasion to share your ideas and speak with colleagues, faculty, friends, or any other interested people. Sharing is important because you can often get very useful advice from like-minded people that helps to clarify your thinking, and it also gives you the opportunity to think about possible supervision and facilities. While the book will not teach you about research methods, it will help you to get your knowledge about relevant research methods into a proposal.

Table i.1   The seven steps in writing a research proposal used in this guide

Chapter	Step	Content
I	Step One: Proposal Preparation	• What is involved in writing a research proposal? • Introducing our researchers and their research topics • Types of proposals • Why proposals fail and succeed
2	Step Two: Background and Justification for the Study	• What is background and justification? • Selective use of the research literature • Reviewing the literature
3	Step Three: Research Approach and Design	• Establishing the research question • Choosing a research approach • Justification of the research approach and methods • Defining and operationalizing concepts for data collection • The 'nuts and bolts' – sampling strategies/data collection/data analysis/limitations/demonstrating rigour
4	Step Four: Capturing Attention – Abstract, Title and Significance	• How to write a detailed abstract that captures attention • Identifying a descriptive, concise and interesting title • How to show that the outcomes will be significant • Structuring for clarity to capture attention • The art of culling words
5	Step Five: Feasibility, Track Record and Teams	• Feasibility • Track record and capability based on research opportunity • Putting together a research team
6	Step Six: Writing an Ethics Proposal	• Ethical practice in research • Research ethics regulatory bodies
7	Step Seven: Writing a Funding Proposal	• Planning ahead • Working with timelines • Guidelines and form fillers • Strategic budgeting • Appendices, letters of support • Committee processes

WHY IS A GUIDE NEEDED FOR WRITING RESEARCH PROPOSALS?

The rigour and clarity of your methods of inquiry are essential to enhance and promote your proposal. Writing a proposal is a problem-solving activity and this step-by-step guide for writing research proposals will assist you to negotiate any problems you encounter. This will save much time in the process, and eventually facilitate committee approval for your study.

As reviewers on research funding and ethical review committees we have often read proposals that are poorly constructed and difficult to understand. Many of these proposals were rejected by the committee. Others were sent back to the applicants for revision which meant delays and extra work for the applicants. It can be very disheartening to have the committee return your proposal with pages of queries. Some students were unaware that they were entitled to get assistance from supervisors while writing their proposal, so it is as well to mention now that writing a proposal is not something you should consider doing on your own. You should be assisted by your supervisor or team and, indeed, it is one of the roles of an academic to provide such assistance.

One way to develop skills in writing clear and concise proposals is to experience what reviewers are looking for by sitting on a review committee. If you can do this then take advantage of the opportunity, although such an invitation is not likely for new researchers. There may be other opportunities for you to familiarize yourself with the research process, and in particular proposals, such as being part of a consortium, or included in some other collaborative research study. Learning from successful researchers can assist you with understanding what is highly regarded by committees. If you are in employment it is useful to make inquiries about ongoing or intended research in your department, and indicate your willingness to be included. This gives you the opportunity to review successful proposals.

'PUT YOURSELF IN THE SHOES' OF THE REVIEW COMMITTEE MEMBER

You are reading a research proposal.

1. What features of a proposal do you consider essential?
2. What would make you reject the proposal?
3. How important would the topic of the proposal be to you?
4. How would you respond to a good research topic but poorly written proposal?

The time that committees will allocate to reviewing your proposal will be limited. It should take you many hours over many weeks to write your proposal and you will become attached to the words that you have written. If the committee is for ethical review or funding, the committee members will have many other proposals to consider. A principal and second reviewer may be allocated to present your application to the committee. They will read your full application, carefully considering the major sections and possibly skim over other sections. They may only be allocated 20 to 30 minutes to present your application to the committee, and the remaining members of the committee may only read the synopsis and major sections of your proposal, meaning that your proposal has to be very clear and convincing. The principal and second reviewer need you to find clear and compelling reasons in your proposal to recommend approval to the committee. These reviewers will have other proposals they have been allocated to present to the committee so they will not have the time, or the inclination, to try to second guess or make assumptions about what you intend in your proposal.

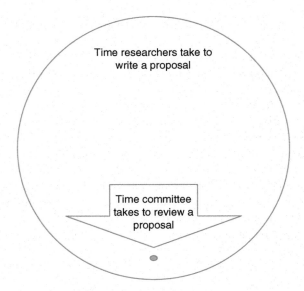

Figure i.1   Time difference to develop and review a research proposal

A recent Australian study found that a new proposal to one of the major health funding agencies, the National Health and Medical Research Council, took on average 38 days of researcher time (Herbert et al., 2013). With the investment of all of this time into a decision that will be made by a committee in 30 to 60 minutes, the proposal needs to be crystal clear and convincing. If we were to draw these time differences it would look something like Figure i.1.

Writing a research proposal for funding is a competitive activity and if the members of the review committee have difficulty in understanding what you are proposing they are likely to lose interest and reject your proposal. If your topic is of interest to the committee, they may return your proposal with many questions requiring clarification. Consider yourself fortunate if you are given this opportunity to address the committee's questions and their offer to allow you to resubmit.

Keep in mind that, in your absence, your proposal is your spokesperson, the vehicle you have authorised to 'speak', on your behalf, to the committee, and the committee is obliged to make a decision about the document they have before them. Your proposal then is your only means at this stage of communicating with the committee, of conveying your ideas, of making a cogent argument for why your topic is worthwhile, relevant and of benefit to people. Your proposal is the means of persuading the committee and gaining their approval, and must therefore, *ipso facto*, be an interesting, clear, readily understood and well written document.

Finally, the time and effort you have put into researching your topic, deciding on a researchable question/statement and completing the research proposal application form must extend to reading the form carefully. Research application forms are all different; there may be some slight but important and notable differences in the information required, and it will save you and the committee a lot of time if you read the form very carefully, and provide the specific information asked for.

This step-by-step approach will enable you to develop a proposal that is written in a clear and logical way so that a committee member reviewing the proposal can easily understand it.

REFERENCES

Herbert, D., Barnett, A., Clarke, P. and Graves, N. (2013) On the time spent preparing grant proposals: an observational study of Australian Researchers. *BMJ Open 2013*;3:e002800 doi:10.1136/bmjopen-2013-002800.

STEP ONE

PROPOSAL PREPARATION

CONTENT

What is involved in writing a research proposal?
Introducing our researchers and their research topics
Types of proposals
Why proposals fail and succeed

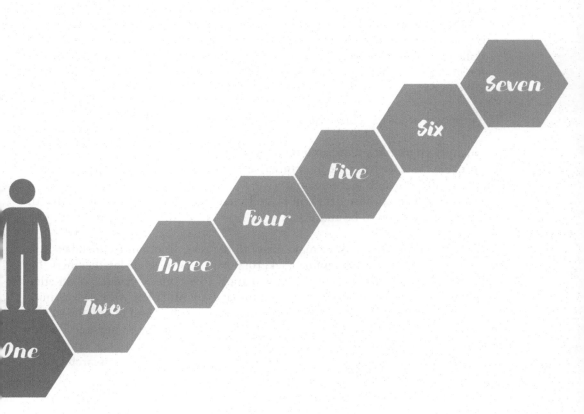

KEY TERMS/ CONCEPTS

- Discipline research conventions
- Problem statement
- Writing pitched to the layperson
- Pre-proposal preparation

WHAT IS INVOLVED IN WRITING A RESEARCH PROPOSAL?

A research proposal is a structured plan, a blue print, of a scientific activity. This means that it needs to build a logical argument that is supported by evidence about the research that you want to conduct. Krathwohl describes the purpose and requirements of a research proposal as:

> an opportunity for you to present your idea and proposed actions for consideration in a shared decision-making situation. You, with all the integrity at your command, are helping those responsible for approving your proposal to see how you view the situation, how the idea fills a need, how it builds on what has been done before, how it will proceed, how you will avoid pitfalls, why pitfalls you have not avoided are not a serious threat, what the study's consequences are likely to be and what significance they are likely to have. It is not a sales job but a carefully prepared, enthusiastic, interestingly written, skilled presentation. Your presentation displays your ability to assemble the foregoing materials into an internally considered chain of reasoning (Krathwohl, 1998, p 65).

The proposal needs to achieve the following:

- identify an important research topic or problem;
- provide evidence from the literature that the study needs to be done;
- establish a research question, and
- set out a plan on how data will be collected and analysed that will enable the research question to be addressed.

The research proposal needs to make sense to the review committee members who may come from different discipline backgrounds as well as some lay members. Lay members are people in the community who apply to become a member of an ethics or research committee. They are required to have no affiliation with the organization to which they have applied for committee membership, and no involvement in any areas of the health sciences, e.g. legal, scientific, medical, or nursing. For this reason the proposal should be written in language that a layperson can understand, stating clearly why the proposal is important and the nature of the research you are planning to undertake.

CONSTRUCTING A RESEARCH ARGUMENT

The language and knowledge domains of disciplines will differ and so the conventions about what is accepted in constructing a research argument in the physical sciences will differ from the social sciences. In quantitative research English is highly conventionalized, and the conventions are fairly consistent across a wide variety of scientific disciplines. This is clearly an advantage for both native and non-native speakers. The conventions involve '(1) structuring arguments and (2) matching linguistic forms to rhetorical purposes. This involves the writer's having to make a series of language choices.' (Weissberg and Buker, 1990: iv). The target audiences in health sciences research are health professionals in your particular discipline and the public. The reasons for following the specific format conventions used in the various disciplines should become clear: in general, the format guides the proposal. In the health sciences, the proposal follows a logical, ordered path, that is, title, abstract, background and justification for the study, research approach and design, significance, feasibility, team track record, ethical and legal issues, and the budget. Language usage should be commensurate with the type of research study proposed. For instance, the use of the first person voice is accepted as a convention in much qualitative social science research. In experimental research, however, the third person voice remains the convention so that the influence of the researcher is seen to be kept at a distance from the research. In experimental research it is required that the researcher exerts no influence on the actual selection of research subjects, beyond setting the inclusion criteria. This is to ensure equal chance of being recruited into the intervention and control arms of a study. In qualitative phenomenological research, however, participants are purposively selected by the researcher because they are likely to be information-rich informants. Even the term 'subjects' is preferred in some disciplines, while in others 'participants' is more accepted. Hence subject recruitment and sampling conventions differ across research disciplines. In a proposal for experimental research a committee would expect to see a hypothesis statement and a research design to test that hypothesis, whereas in a qualitative social science proposal the committee would expect to see a research question and a research design that would add insight to answer that question. You should be aware of the language and research design conventions of the disciplines that are dealt with by the committee to whom you are sending the proposal so that you know which conventions will be accepted and which will be questioned.

TOP TIP

Know the accepted conventions of your discipline.

A TASK THAT IS MORE THAN JUST WRITING THE WORDS: PRE-PROPOSAL PREPARATION

Writing a research proposal can be a considerable task especially if it is for one of the main national granting agencies, such as the National Institute of Health (USA), the Medical Research Council (United Kingdom), the National Health and Medical Research Council (Australia), or the Health Research Council (New Zealand). These applications, with attachments that contain the curriculum vitae of each member of the research team, can run into more than 100 pages, and so putting together such a proposal will be demanding and time-consuming. The application for a small grant, a higher degree proposal or an ethics application will not be as big an undertaking as this, but you will still need to do your preparatory work and so allow plenty of time to develop the proposal before the submission date. This is the pre-proposal preparation.

As most research proposals involve a team and will require access to participants or to existing data, preparatory work will need to be undertaken before the proposal is written. Depending upon the nature of your study, decisions about participants and other people, possible designs and sites will have to be considered. If your study is for a higher degree, you (and your supervisor) will be making decisions about the feasibility of access to participants (hospital, residential care, community), sites, the study design (qualitative, quantitative, focus groups, mixed methods), costs, and so on. If generating a team for the study is required, this will also necessitate accessing suitable co-researchers and exploring the feasibility with them of undertaking the project. All this information will eventually be part of your proposal.

 # READ-REFLECT-RESPOND 1.1

You are working in the Department of Health and have access to a large quantity of epidemiological data for the city you live in. There is research evidence to show that the incidence of smoking in school children aged 15–17 years is increasing. You would like to conduct a study to investigate the smoking and smoking cessation rates of boys and girls in this age group. There are two people in your workplace who would be appropriate members of a team.

What preparatory work would you have to undertake before you begin writing a proposal?

ONCE YOU HAVE MADE THE DECISION TO PROCEED

After you have undertaken your initial preparation and made the decision to proceed you should remember that a proposal is a piece of technical writing, but like all writing, the product will improve with subsequent drafts. Prepare yourself and your team for the time that it will take to write and review a number of drafts before the final proposal is submitted.

INTRODUCING OUR RESEARCHERS AND THEIR RESEARCH TOPICS

You will now be introduced to two hypothetical researchers, Natasha and Liang, who have each identified a topic or problem in their respective disciplines that they want to research. With your help in using this Guide, Natasha and Liang will develop their proposals in steps through the activities provided in each chapter. You can complete the activities for both Natasha and Liang as you are likely to learn more in doing this, or you can simply complete the activity for one of them depending upon which one is of interest to you.

NATASHA

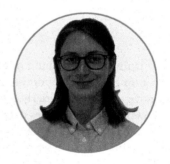

Natasha is a midwife of 10 years standing. She works in the maternity section of a large city hospital. Natasha's duties include working in the antenatal clinic of the hospital assisting with registration of women in the first trimester of their pregnancy. Natasha assists the women in completing a questionnaire about their current physical and emotional health status. During this activity Natasha had noticed that similar issues were identified by the women. For example, they complained about feeling ambivalent, lacking control over their symptoms, feeling stressed and anxious, vomiting, experiencing overwhelming fatigue, nausea, not feeling very optimistic about the pregnancy, and generally becoming fearful.

The problem that natasha sees and wants to research

Natasha's major interest in her midwifery work is trying to find a way to assist the women with their feelings of passivity and anxiety in the first trimester by helping them identify their coping strategies. She is hoping that by identifying the women's perceptions of their anxiety and also their strengths, she will help them to cope with their anxiety and fear.

Natasha completed a Master of Nursing (Research) 4 years ago. She has completed a unit in qualitative research and a unit in quantitative research methods. She now wants to enrol for a PhD programme at the university in order to investigate pregnant women's strategies of coping and their impact on fear and anxiety in the first trimester of their pregnancy. She would like to use a qualitative research approach and conduct in-depth interviews with 40 women.

LIANG

Liang completed his PhD four years ago in which he wrote an epidemiological thesis into the presentation of older people in General Practice who have co-morbid chronic illness. (General Practice may be called Family Practice, Primary Care or Community Medicine in some other countries.) He found a high prevalence of people with a chronic physical condition, such as diabetes or heart disease, who were also depressed. One of the recommendations that he made at the conclusion of his study was that further research was needed into the capacity of General Practice to provide treatments for people with co-morbidities.

The problem that Liang sees and wants to research

During his PhD, Liang noted that the systems used in General Practice seemed best set up for short appointments to deal with one problem at a time. He also observed, in the case of his elderly mother who has diabetes, that when she attends her GP, she receives good diabetes care, but no one asks her how she is coping emotionally with her diabetes and managing her condition in her daily life.

Liang has just been awarded a 4 year post-doctoral fellowship at the Primary Health Care Research Institute and he would like to continue his research into co-morbid chronic illness. As a quantitative researcher he would like to test an intervention that could improve the system of care for people with co-morbid conditions in General Practice. Liang has read some of the literature that proposes that the role of nurses be expanded to work in a team with GPs in a more systematic management of care.

NOTE: *The problem that Liang is wanting to research is based on a real study that has been adapted with permission from the Australian TrueBlue trial (Morgan et al., 2013).*

Not to be overlooked in the early stages of thinking about your research topic, and about writing a research proposal, is the importance of discussing your idea with relevant people. In Natasha's case it would be prudent, in the first instance, to discuss her idea, and the feasibility of doing the study, with the nurse manager in charge of the antenatal clinic. If the nurse manager is supportive, Natasha would need to negotiate time (leave) to conduct the study, and possibly a replacement in the antenatal clinic, with the Director of Nursing. Finally, Natasha may also need to approach a midwife knowledgeable in her topic area for supervision.

For Liang, a discussion with experts in the management of chronic illness in General Practice could inform him about any other studies in this area and whether his study would be worthwhile. Discussion with senior people in peak General Practice and nursing organizations would help Liang to determine the likelihood of general practitioners and nurses participating in the study. Finally, Liang would need to discuss with the Director of the Primary Health Care Research Institute the support that would be available for this study during his post-doctoral fellowship with the Institute.

The next activity asks you to respond to the research examples that we have provided from Natasha and Liang. Activities related to Natasha or Liang will appear in each step. Completing these activities will give you practice in writing the sections of a research proposal in stepwise manner. We have provided our responses to these activities at the end of each step so that you can compare your response with ours. After each practice activity you are then asked to work on the similar step of your own research proposal.

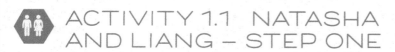

ACTIVITY 1.1 NATASHA AND LIANG – STEP ONE

This activity is the same for both Natasha and Liang. You can complete the activity for both or either one. If you do both we suggest you complete them as separate activities.

1. Write a working problem statement or research question that Natasha and Liang could use as a starting point for discussion.
2. It would be wise for Natasha and Liang to discuss their research question with appropriate people. List at least three different types of people that Natasha and Liang should approach and what she/he should discuss with them.
3. What skills and resources are Natasha and Liang likely to have that will enable and/or limit their proposed research?
4. What resources should Natasha and Liang acquire to deal with these limits and so enable the research?

See our response on p. 14.

Having completed the practice activity it is now time to work on Step One of your proposal.

ACTIVITY 1.2 YOUR PROPOSAL – STEP ONE

1. In order to have a discussion with a colleague or your supervisor about what you want to research it will be helpful to write a few paragraphs of 300–400 words to introduce yourself and the problem that you think needs researching. Before writing these paragraphs it would be wise to do a scan of the literature to identify what research has already been done on this topic. This will help you to form some early ideas about gaps and methodological issues in published research and so the need for such a study.
2. Approach three different types of people to discuss your idea.
3. Describe the skills and resources you have that will enable and limit your proposed research.
4. What resources would you need in addition to those you already have to deal with these limits and so enable the research? Make a note of these as this will help you in Step Five on team track record.
5. Make a note of your response to points three and four as these will help you later in Step Five on feasibility and team track record.
6. Having canvassed your idea and considered your skills and resources, you now need to decide whether to proceed with the development of a proposal. Use the checklist below to help you decide.

CHECKLIST:

- Evidence from the literature about your research topic/problem.
- Identification of knowledge gaps; omissions; methodological issues in the existing literature.
- Does the research topic/problem align with the university/health service/funding agency research priorities? (See Step 7 on how to write a funding proposal.)
- Researcher skills and resources available.

TYPES OF PROPOSALS

You have now found a problem that you wish to research. You have conducted a preliminary reading of the literature and you have discussed your idea with the pertinent people in your faculty or health service to canvas their opinion on whether your topic is appropriate, relevant, feasible and researchable.

You are now faced with a research proposal format. The format of a proposal depends upon which committee the proposal is for: an application to a university higher degrees committee; a site specific assessment application to the management of the organization in which the study is planned; an application to an ethics review board; or a funding application. Each type of proposal has a purpose which is described in Table 1.1. and these will be examined in detail in later steps. Time spent reading, very carefully, the proposal pro forma requirements is time well spent and advantageous both from your perspective and that of the committee.

Table 1.1   Types and purpose of research proposals

Proposal	Purpose
Higher Degrees Committee	Show the potential student's academic capability to identify a research problem and propose a logical study that will address this problem. The committee will want to be confident that a student has had the prior education required to become a higher degree student, that the study can be supervised, and that the proposed project can be achieved as a higher degree study.
Site Specific Assessment	Consideration by the management of a site (organization) that the proposed research can be accommodated within the current activities and demands on the site and also that the research is not contrary to the interests of the organization, the staff, and clients.
Ethical Review Committee	Approve only research that meets the established ethical standards and that the benefits to the public of the research outweigh any cost or burden on participants.
Funding Committee	Determine that the proposed research is in line with the funding priorities set by the committee and that the best proposals are approved within the limits of the funding available to the committee.

READ–REFLECT–RESPOND 1.2

'IT TAKES MORE THAN GRANT WRITING TO WIN A GRANT'

Brainstorm alone or with a colleague what might be meant by this statement. See our response in the appendix.

Not only will a proposal differ according to the committee to which it is sent, but the content and logical basis of the proposal can differ in various disciplines, such as between the physical and earth sciences, humanities, medical and health sciences and social sciences. This text relates to proposals in the health sciences that require the collection of original data from the field. While there is no specific formula for research proposals, in general there is a stepped structure that will facilitate and guide a researcher's thinking. Ultimately, these steps do much to ensure a clear, concise and logical description of the topic that you wish to research.

WHY PROPOSALS FAIL AND SUCCEED

A proposal may fail to get through a committee approval process if it is poorly written and argued, as we have explained. The National Institute of Nursing Research (undated) has categorized common mistakes in research proposal development under four headings (Table 1.2):

Table 1.2   Common mistakes in research proposals

Aim	• too ambitious
	• unfocused
	• unclear (future) direction
Significance	• no advance on knowledge (beyond this case)
	• lacks compelling rationale
	• no impact
Design	• too much detail/too little detail
	• feasibility not shown
	• lack of expertise in the team (content &/or method)
	• the study does not answer the research question
Environment	• little institutional support
	• insufficient resources

As a way of helping applications to ensure that proposals are approved, the US Grantsmanship Center (undated) has described the five elements that can make or break a research proposal and we recommend that you keep these points in mind.

1. Identify a significant problem with a focused and manageable research question.
2. Define outcomes that are realistic and attainable.
3. Describe methods to achieve the outcomes that show the logical sequence of ideas.
4. Establish your and your team's credibility (track record).
5. Identify future funding sources, or at least what future work this research will lead to.

PROPOSAL WRITING: AN ESSENTIAL RESEARCH SKILL

Proposal writing is an essential skill and is the medium through which you sell your ideas. This involves writing for impact. Writing skills develop accumulatively – the more you write, the more skilled you are likely to become. Good writing also requires an understanding of grammar, clarity, and a sound knowledge of your topic based on your review of the literature. Peha (1995) describes 'good' writing as 'Ideas that are interesting and important; organization that is logical and effective; voice that is individual and appropriate; word choice that is specific and memorable; sentence fluency that is smooth and expressive, and conventions that are correct and communicative.' Drawing a concept map to clarify your concepts of interest is a helpful exercise, and this is discussed in detail in Step 2.

Achieving success with a research proposal involves competition with others. If seeking to enrol in a PhD, there will only be a limited number of places in a higher degree programme, or if the proposal is for funding, the success rate is rarely higher than 30% approval. This means that your proposal has to be good (that is, it has to meet the criteria discussed previously); however, there is a good chance that your proposal will not be successful on the first application or at least be sent back for further work.

WRITING FOR THE LAYPERSON

We suggest you write your proposal at the level of a layperson, avoiding overuse of technical language, jargon and colloquialisms. This is because many committee members may not be experts, or even knowledgeable, in the field of study or in the method that you are proposing. While the text should make use of appropriate technical language, this should be used judiciously and explained in a way that the layperson can follow.

Make sure that you use facts to convince the reader that your logic is sound, and be specific rather than make sweeping generalizations. Too often broad statements are made such as 'there is a paucity of research about this topic', rather than adding a few sentences that detail what research has been done and what still needs to be done. Similarly, be specific in referring to your research approach, rather than simply describing it as being 'qualitative', for example, as it could leave the committee guessing unless you specify exactly which qualitative approach you are using, e.g. grounded theory, phenomenology or ethnography.

You can help the reader follow your proposal if you construct your argument in a way that takes them through your logic in a step-by-step manner. The reader should not have to jump around between sections in order to make sense of what you are proposing. You should also be consistent in the terms you use. For instance, it would confuse the reader if you referred to a 'focus group' in the synopsis section, but then later referred to this as a 'workshop' in the research plan section. Other terms often used interchangeably and inconsistently are 'research participant' and 'research inform-ant'. This should be avoided and you should also be consistent in the way that you lay out the text. For instance, the order in which you describe data collection strategies pertinent to each research objective should be consistent with the order in which you have listed these objectives. Use headings, subheadings, bold and italicized text, bullet points and diagrams as these can help the reader to follow the steps in your logic.

Our final tip in writing for success is to make the proposal look good. Poor for-matting, spelling errors and a lack of white space on the page (trying to cram too much in) give readers a poor impression of your work. Text formatting can be a nightmare when using the templates provided by funding agencies so it is worth sorting out how to work with the required template well before the proposal sub-mission date. We will come back to this in Step 7 on funding proposals.

THINK STRATEGICALLY ABOUT WHICH COMMITTEE IS RIGHT FOR YOU

In seeking to sell your research idea, it is also worth considering which committee to target. You may have a great idea, say to research chronic disease management, but it would be fruitless to submit a higher degree proposal for such a study to a faculty of engineering, or a grant agency that only funds basic research, rather than applied health services research. So to be successful your proposal needs to:

- show clear evidence of feasibility regarding all aspects of the research design;
- be well written to sell the idea;
- be sent to the right committee.

CONCLUSION

This chapter has alerted you to the need to undertake your pre-proposal preparation. This involves discussion with relevant key people prior to making the decision to proceed with the written work that is involved. You have now completed the first exercises in the Guide related to identifying your research problem and your first preparatory steps.

In describing the amount of work and the pitfalls in writing a proposal about your research idea, it would be remiss of us to leave you with the impression that writing a proposal is little more than an onerous activity, no matter how dedicated and committed you are to your research idea. What you will discover is the thrill and excitement you experience, when, after your many hours of thorough and careful proposal preparation and submission to the relevant committee, you receive a letter from the committee advising you of your success.

The next step is writing a compelling background and justification for the study.

REVISION

Below you will find five statements related to the content of this step. Indicate whether you believe each statement to be true or false. The answers are given on p. 15.

1. It is a good idea to share your research interests with like-minded people.

   T/F

2. If your research topic is good the research committee will accept it.

   T/F

3. You should assume that you should write a proposal without assistance from a supervisor or fellow team member.

   T/F

4. Pre-proposal preparation will identify any issues requiring clarification prior to writing your proposal.

   T/F

5. It is unusual for a proposal to be funded at the first submission.

   T/F

REFERENCES

Krathwohl, D.R. (1998) *Methods of Educational and Social Science Research: An integrated approach*. New York: Longman.

Morgan, M., Coates, M., Dunbar, J., Reddy, P., Schlicht, K. and Fuller, J. (2013) The TrueBlue model of collaborative care using practice nurses as case managers for depression alongside diabetes or heart disease. *BMJ Open*, 3(1) doi: 10.1136/bmjopen-2012-002171.

National Institute of Nursing Research. (www.ninr.nih.gov/Training/Grantsmanship). [last accessed 27 August 2017]

The Grantsmanship Center. (www.tgci.com). [last accessed 27 August 2017]

Peha, S. (1995) Teaching That Makes Sense. (www.ttms.org). [last accessed 27 August 2017]

Weissberg, R. and Buker, S. (1990) *Writing up research*. Englewood Cliffs, NJ: Prentice Hall Regents.

ADDITIONAL READING

There are a huge number of internet accessible resources on the writing of research proposals. We have listed just a few that we have found helpful and that we specifically used in this first step.

- The Grantsmanship Center

  A US-based centre that provides material and training in writing successful grant proposals for funding (www.tgci.com). [last accessed 27 August 2017]

- The National Institute of Nursing Research (NINR)

  An Institute within the US National Institute of Health. The NINR promote improvements in health care through research and research training (www.ninr.nih.gov). [last accessed 27 August 2017]

- How not to kill a grant application

  (http://blog.globalacademyjobs.com/how-not-to-kill-a-grant-application).[last accessed 27 August 2017]

ANSWERS TO ACTIVITIES

ACTIVITY 1.1

NATASHA

Q1. What are the physiological and psychological changes that women report during the first 13 weeks of pregnancy?

Q2. Natasha should approach the Head of the Midwifery Unit to discuss with them and also colleagues whether they consider this an important problem and, if so, the feasibility of conducting the research in the Unit. Natasha should discuss her idea with a senior research midwife at the hospital to see if they can offer field supervision to her during her data collection. She should also find a suitable academic midwife interested in the topic for academic supervision. Natasha would have already read some literature to establish the need for her proposed study. She would have identified clearly the gaps and omissions of some previous studies. Finally, Natasha would need to find out from the Director of Nursing at the hospital if she would be granted leave (either part-time or full-time) to study for a PhD.

Natasha could also look for agencies prepared to fund women's studies as well as enquire at the hospital and university who may provide scholarships. She could access scholarship details from the various agencies in order to see their proposal formats, guidelines and submission dates.

Q3. Natasha is a registered midwife. She completed two research units (quantitative and qualitative research methods) during her Master of Nursing degree through coursework. She has a good grasp of grounded theory and would like to use this research approach for her proposed study. While she has conducted limited research under supervision for her Master's programme, Natasha would require close supervision from a knowledgeable academic with an interest in her topic.

Q4. Natasha should review her interviewing skills with a midwifery academic. She should also review and understand very clearly (although she has conducted a small study previously) the procedures involved in a grounded theory approach.

LIANG

Q1. Can a system of chronic disease care planning be implemented in General Practice that leads to positive client outcomes? Would the system be feasible within the role and skill capacity of nurses working in General Practice and within the current levels of funding available for General Practice services?

Q2. Liang should talk to an academic GP and academic nurse with a background in primary care to ask them if they know of any research that has been done on this topic, and their opinion on what else needs to be done. He should meet with the local representative of the GP or General Practice Nursing Organization to see if they think the idea has merit and, if so, would they support him as 'field advisors' in developing a proposal. He should meet with the head of his Institute to ascertain if this topic would be a priority and if it would be supported by the Institute.

Q3. Liang clearly has a research background that is relevant to this topic. He is located in a Primary Health Care Research Institute and so his work environment is suitable. Having a 4 year post-doctoral fellowship may provide Liang with the time to undertake this project although this may depend on what else is expected of him during the fellowship.

Q4. Liang has the necessary research skills given that he has completed an epidemiological PhD. He has quantitative skills and so should be able to conduct an intervention trial. However, he may not currently have the theoretical or methodological knowledge and skills needed in organizational systems and health services research.

READ–REFLECT–RESPOND 1.2

While the proposal is the formal documentation of the research plan, the development of such a plan and successful approval of the plan will depend on much more: it also involves the development of research networks, a research track record and, most importantly, a research programme over a career that starts with smaller exploratory studies leading up to larger explanatory studies.

There is a period of pre-proposal preparation and a series of decisions to be made prior to writing a proposal that include:

- determining that you have a worthwhile research question or problem. This may involve talking with colleagues and experts in the field and will certainly require a preliminary reading of the research literature;
- getting a research team together;
- ensuring that you can get access to participants or to data to undertake a study;
- deciding the level at which to pitch a proposal based on track record, team capacity, access to data and availability of resources, such as funds;
- framing the first draft of an operational research question.

REVISION STATEMENTS

1. T
2. F
3. F
4. T
5. T

STEP TWO

BACKGROUND AND JUSTIFICATION FOR THE STUDY

CONTENT

What is background and justification?

Selective use of the research literature

Reviewing the literature

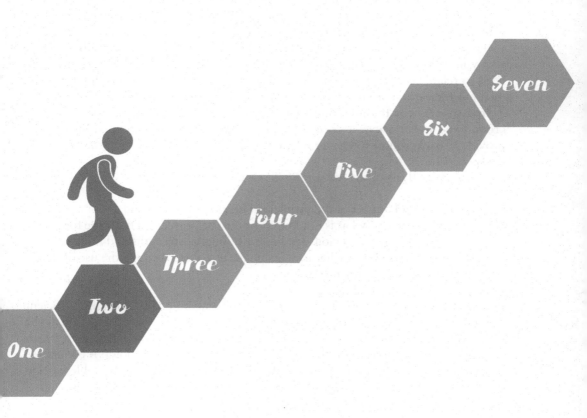

KEY TERMS/CONCEPTS

- Justification
- Topic gap
- Method gap
- Theoretical or conceptual framework
- Concept mapping
- PICO question
- Key search terms
- Grey literature
- Black literature

WHAT IS BACKGROUND AND JUSTIFICATION?

This chapter will guide you on how to write a careful and economical literature review to provide a background to the research topic/problem and a justification for the study. The background of a study provides a review of the specific topic being investigated, and importantly includes relevant research studies about this topic. The purpose of the background is to indicate your familiarity with the research field of your topic. This will include the identification and critique of the different methodologies in the studies you have quoted in order to provide evidence of what previous studies have achieved and where gaps exist.

These gaps are the basis and justification for your research study, in other words, why you believe it is important to conduct your study. By justification we mean the need to relate your proposed study to what is already known about the topic and then put forward an argument about what needs further investigation.

In research, it is the literature that is considered as the evidence for this background and justification. A critical analysis of this literature is needed in order to provide a background to the problem and also as justification for the proposed study.

A critical analysis of the literature will establish the following:

1. The extent and impact of the problem. **This is the background.**
2. What is known and what is not known about the problem. **This is the topic gap.**
3. The methods used in previous studies including the strengths and limitations of these methods and also what insights might be gained through the use of different methods. **This is the method gap.**

By describing the extent and impact of the problem, you are establishing sufficient background for the reader to see the relative importance of the problem, such as the proportion of population affected (extent is large or small), and the degree to which the problem has an impact on the lives of those affected (high or low). A committee that is considering the approval of a study will want to know that the problem being investigated is of sufficient importance to justify the effort required to conduct the study. For instance, a study into vaginal thrush may be considered important because it affects a large proportion of women (around 75% over a lifetime), rather than because of the impact on a woman's life, where the uncomplicated symptoms can be easily treated. Here the extent of the problem is relatively high but the impact may be considered as relatively low. A study into chronic childhood leukaemia may be considered important, not because of the proportion of children affected, as this is a rare disease, but because it can be debilitating to individuals over the long term and can lead to death in 20% to 40% of those affected. Here the extent of the problem is relatively low, but the impact is relatively high.

Establishing the importance of a problem is, however, not sufficient justification for a study to proceed. A study needs to add some new knowledge and so address one of the gaps. A study can address a **topic gap** by asking a new research question, or even by asking a follow-on question, for example this occurs when a large study is proposed based on the findings of a previous pilot study. A study can address a **method gap** by using different methods to research the same problem in order to overcome limitations or omissions in the previous methods. For instance, an ethnographic qualitative study of illicit drug use by teenagers could explore their drug use influences and motivations in a way that would not be possible through a large population-based survey that was designed to establish prevalence of use.

When analysing the literature on previous research studies, there will be variation regarding aims and objectives, and sample and data collection and analysis, even within the same type of studies. These differences should be carefully considered because they will have an effect on the previous findings and, consequently, what can be said about what is already known, and what is not known. Sometimes it is simply that the findings from previous studies are inconclusive, and this therefore warrants further studies to see if more conclusive findings can be ascertained. For example, Harrison and Gibbons (2013, p 396) justified their study about student perceptions of concept maps on the basis that the literature revealed only 'partial glimpses of what students experience when they learn to use concept maps'. The authors argued that a study was needed to obtain a more comprehensive picture before they felt they could fully implement concept maps into their nursing programme.

SELECTIVE USE OF THE RESEARCH LITERATURE

It is likely that a large body of literature relevant to your topic will be identified. While you should read extensively, a careful, focused search and a critical reading of the literature will be needed for your proposal, so that you can argue the need for your study. The space allocated in a proposal template for the background and justification may allow only a few pages for this, and so this section needs to be focused, concise and clear in making the argument.

ESTABLISHING THE GAPS

Your reading of the literature should be carefully planned and ordered in relation to the specific concepts you wish to explore. Above all, a literature review is an evaluative report of your sources of information. An analysis of the literature requires critical reading and critical analysis to ensure that a cogent argument can be made about why it is important to conduct your study. It is important to identify studies with research designs similar to yours (e.g. qualitative, quantitative, mixed methods) and also studies that have different research designs. A critical analysis of the studies can identify possible problems associated with methodology, the theoretical framework, participant recruitment, inclusion and exclusion criteria, study site, research design, nature of informed consent, and other ethical issues. These are all factors which may increase the difficulty of making comparisons between studies.

How well you critically analyse the literature to highlight topic and method gaps is, to use a military analogy, the major weapon in your arsenal. Your critique of the literature must convince the committee why your research design and methods will provide the missing meaningful information about the topic. A critical analysis of the studies, and clearly distinguishing differences between studies, should convince the committee that the study, in the form in which you are presenting it, is important (and why), has not been done before, and that the results will enhance the current knowledge base of the topic.

CAUTION

We have discussed the need to provide a justification for a study in the background section of a research proposal. It is important here to explain the difference between the justification (the significance of a study) and innovation. To recap, the significance of a research problem relates to the importance of undertaking the study, why it is needed, how you intend to address the missing gaps, and why you (and/or your team) are qualified to address the problem. There are numerous definitions of 'innovation', but generally innovation refers to a new product, idea or process which introduces a significant positive change that adds value to the organization. An example of innovation, of introducing a new product or idea, will illustrate the point. The innovation is a framework to understand the appropriation of IT as an innovation within early childhood education: the three perspectives of innovation are: an individual, a structuralist and an interactive process perspective (Plumb and Kautz, 2014).

Proposal templates often have separate sections for these different concepts and poor applications will repeat the same information. We will deal with significance in Step 4, but suffice to say here that significance is about expanding the argument on importance in order to examine for whom it is important, that is, whether it is important for government, for particular organizations, for sections of the population, etc. This can be done by situating the problem within the context of national policies, and detailing how the study findings may help solve the problems described in these policies.

USING A THEORETICAL FRAMEWORK

It is likely that, during your review of the literature, you will make a decision about whether or not to use a theoretical framework or conceptual model to guide your study. A theoretical framework informs the research problem and embraces all aspects of the study logic. The study logic is the sequence of the argument from which the existing knowledge about the problem is understood, that leads to a new research question being asked, for which relevant study aims and objectives are set, and that the data collection and analysis approach proposed will enable the research question to be answered.

Distinguishing between theoretical framework of content and theory of method

It is important to distinguish between the theoretical framework of content and the theory of the method. The theory of the method is the methodology, which is about the research approach most appropriate to answer the research question: this is dealt with in Step 3. The theoretical framework of content is about concepts that we use to understand the component parts of the problem, and this is described below.

Using an explicit theoretical framework of content will ensure that you make it clear to the reader how you are building on existing knowledge and what is new about your proposed study.

Using a theoretical framework (or conceptual model) helps you to consider what aspects of the problem your study will deal with, and this gives your study a direction. The theoretical framework is also used as a basis for the discussion of your findings about what is new, and this is often called the 'so what' aspect of a study. Gray and Sockolow (2016) state that 'contributing to health informatics research means using conceptual models that are integrative and explain the research in terms of the two broad domains of health science and information science'. The authors concede however, that it may be difficult for novice researchers to find examples and guidelines to assist them in working with integrative conceptual models. Another example comes from Sercekus and Mete (2010) who used the Roy adaptation model to assess the effects of antenatal education on the maternal prenatal and post-partum adaptation of 120 nulliparous women (women who have never borne a child). In general, it is often useful to embed your study into some kind of framework to assist with the clarification and explication of concepts and their relationships.

There are many websites that provide detailed information about theoretical frameworks, including the following two examples:

- University of Southern California Library Research Guides. Organizing your social sciences research paper: theoretical framework. http://libguides.usc.edu/writingguide/theoreticalframework.
- Scribbr. The theoretical framework of a dissertation: what and how. www.scribbr.com/dissertation/the-theoretical-framework-of-a-dissertation-what-and-how.

CONCEPT MAPPING

Concept mapping is one way to develop your theoretical framework of content. The place to start with this is the working problem statement and study title that were developed as a part of Step One, 'finding the research problem'. However, this working problem statement and title will most likely change as you begin to review the literature. You should be open-minded, flexible and prepared to modify or adjust your thinking as you read the research literature.

According to Harrison and Gibbons (2013, p 395), 'Constructing concept maps requires reflection, creativity, and insight, all of which are key skills associated with critical thinking'.

NATASHA'S CONCEPT MAP

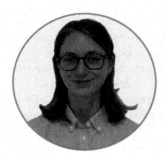

Natasha's working title was 'An investigation into pregnant women's experiences of ambivalence, anxiety and fears in the first trimester of pregnancy, and how they cope with their feelings.'

Even before conducting her literature review, Natasha identified many concepts of interest relating to her topic. She first listed these without looking for any relationship between them.

Initial concept list

- Experience of pregnancy
- Attitude towards pregnancy, i.e. regards it as a sick role or well state
- Sources of information about pregnancy
- Support, living conditions – alone, with partner, with parents
- Coping strategies
- General health prior to becoming pregnant
- Pregnancy planned/unplanned
- Attitude towards the physical and emotional changes
- Locus of control, external or internal
- Experience of physical, emotional and cognitive changes
- Pregnancy as 'crisis', an upsetting, inconvenient time
- Financial security

She then drew a map with all the concepts. Where it made sense she identified those concepts that were related. After this she began the process of eliminating less related concepts and concentrated on those remaining. She continued to look for connections, similarities and differences between concepts. The result was the identification of six concepts which Natasha felt were most closely related to her objectives (Figure 2.1). This concept map will probably change as Natasha completes her literature review.

Natasha identified six major concepts:

- 'living' the pregnancy: experiences of anxiety and/or fear;
- attitude to pregnancy;
- locus of control;
- support; emotional and financial (from partner, parents, friends, professionals, others);
- coping strategies;
- pregnancy planned/unplanned.

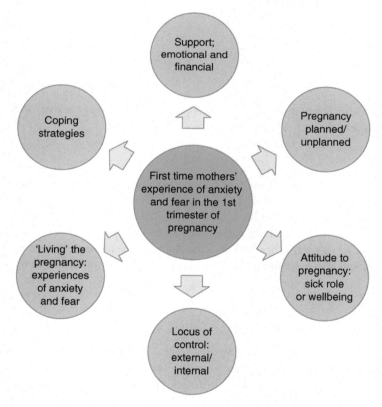

Figure 2.1   Concept map for first time mothers' experience of anxiety and fear in the first trimester of pregnancy

Following the identification of the concepts in your study, in most cases you will need to operationally define them, even if they have been defined in previous studies. You will need to define what you mean when you refer to a concept so that the reader is clear about what you are referring to and, also, that you are clear about what you are collecting data on. However, this rule of operationally defining concepts does not apply across all exploratory type studies. For example, even though concepts like anxiety and fear may have been previously defined in studies on pregnant women, Natasha does not want to impose any particular definition on anxiety and fear, or begin her fieldwork with any preconceptions about the nature of what anxiety and fear mean to the women. Rather she wants to explore, through in-depth interviews, and through the narrative the women provide, what anxiety and fear mean to them and so allow the meanings of their unique experiences to emerge from the data.

In Natasha's concept map (Figure 2.1) the six concepts sit separately around the research working title, and without links between them. The resulting map is like a star diagram. Another researcher's concept map of a similar topic might look quite different and one would expect differences in researcher interests.

TOP TIP

Creating a concept map for your research idea is a worthwhile activity in the early stages of idea development.

In a topic like Natasha's, you may find many other important concepts that interest you in addition to the ones that Natasha has identified. Trying to incorporate all the concepts into your framework would make a study unwieldy. Writing your particular concepts onto a concept map will make it easier for you to identify the concepts that are connected or related to each other, and so limit the number to be examined in one study. This method will also help you to focus, and provide clarity and direction to your study.

LIANG'S CONCEPT MAP

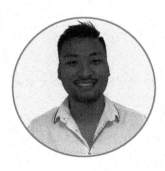

Liang wants to test the implementation of a system of team-based chronic disease care planning in General Practice that leads to positive outcomes for patients with co-morbid depression and diabetes and/or heart disease. He would like to determine if a system would be feasible within the role and skill capacity of nurses working in a General Practice team and within the current levels of funding available for General Practice services.

Liang first brainstormed the following list of concepts that he considered relevant to this topic.

Initial concept list

- Patient with chronic disease
- Co-morbidity
- Collaborative practice
- General Practice Team
    - GP
    - Nurse
- System of care
    - Care planning
    - Staff roles
    - Best-practice protocols
    - Skills development
    - Care continuity and coordination
    - Patient chronic disease management support
- Funding

He then put these concepts together in a map as a way of showing how the concepts were related and which seemed to be the core concepts.

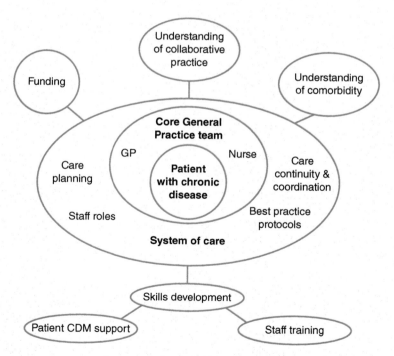

Figure 2.2   Concept map for a team-based intervention that could improve the system of care for people with co-morbid conditions in General Practice

Stating assumptions

The assumptions made about a study need to be stated. The assumptions are views that the researcher takes for granted, whether based on their own thinking or derived from the literature, and these should be clearly stated in order that the reader can view the proposed study in the framework of the researcher's study design. Specificity and clarity about concepts and assumptions regarding the topic would prevent the committee having to ask for clarification and possibly delay the progress of the study.

READ–REFLECT–RESPOND 2.1

NATASHA'S ASSUMPTIONS

Notwithstanding Israeloff's (1985:14) description of pregnancy as ' ... like adolescence – a circum-scribed, transitional period riddled with ambivalence, a set-apart, self-conscious time ... occasioning great shows of opinion and theory, but which finally must be simply endured', Natasha's view of pregnancy is that pregnancy is normal and natural while acknowledging that the disorders of pregnancy – vomiting, nausea, fatigue – in general, are annoying rather than disabling, are of limited duration, and should be expected and accepted as part of the pregnant condition. She considers the women to be 'well'; their condition one of *wellbeing*.

    Natasha's reluctance to impose a definition on any of her concepts is illustrated by the example of at least three ways in which the concept of *wellbeing* has been defined. If you conduct an internet search on *wellbeing*, you will find a variety of definitions to choose from such as the following:

- A good or satisfactory condition of existence, a state characterised by health, happiness, and prosperity. www.dictionary.com/browse/well-being
- *Wellbeing* is not just the absence of disease or illness. It is a complex combination of a person's physical, mental, emotional and social health factors. www.betterhealth.vic.gov.au/health/health-yliving/wellbeing
- Contrary to popular belief, *wellbeing* is different from happiness. Happiness can come and go in a moment whereas *wellbeing* is a more stable state (Raibley, 2012).

   1.   If you were Natasha, which definition of *wellbeing* would you choose from the three listed above? Give reasons for your choice.
   2.   If you think it is needed, write or adapt your own definition of *wellbeing* that would best suit the problem that Natasha is exploring.

There are many more definitions of *wellbeing*. Your particular philosophy about what you think constitutes *wellbeing* is important because your definition is what will provide the framework for your study. For example, if *wellbeing* were defined as the absence of disease or illness, it may be too rigid a definition to reflect how some people with diseases view themselves, in other words, how incapacitated by their disease they perceive themselves to be. They may question why a person with diabetes or heart disease cannot feel a sense of wellbeing if their particular condition is under control and they are living what they consider to be a satisfying, pain-free and healthy life.

REVIEWING THE LITERATURE
REFINING CONCEPTS INTO KEY TERMS AND A RESEARCH QUESTION

Once you have mapped your topic of interest, choosing key terms will assist in limiting and also refining the extent of your literature search. For example, let's assume you are interested in investigating broad concepts like *culture, suffering, cultural attitudes* and *cultural beliefs*. Does *culture* refer to a specific ethnic group? Are you using western culture as a category in the conceptual framework? Are *attitudes* individual or personal attitudes or group attitudes? Identify precisely what *beliefs* you are investigating. Are they spiritual or religious beliefs or beliefs about health and wellbeing? Does *suffering* refer to physical pain or mental suffering? This is simply an example of the clarity of purpose that is required when embarking on a literature search. Refining and limiting your concepts and related key terms will save you much time and help you crystallize your thinking.

You will find hundreds of articles on these concepts, and they in turn may include a large variety of additional concepts. Apart from key terms like *culture, suffering, cultural attitudes* and *cultural beliefs,* you would need to identify as concisely and clearly as possible which specific group, in terms of ethnicity, education, gender, age, presence or absence of existing medical condition, cognition, ability to speak and understand a specific language, you are wanting to investigate.

Because of the large volume of research literature, it is best to set a restricted or limited question initially that will focus your search only on the concepts and key terms that you have specified. If you find that a restrictive search produces very few articles then you can broaden the focus by altering or removing key terms that might be limiting the focus.

The mnemonic PICO has been developed to help researchers frame a searchable question for a literature review. While originally developed to search for evidence from clinical trials, the mnemonic can be adapted as PICo to suit observational as well as qualitative studies (Joanna Briggs Institute, 2014).

Table 2.1   Components of the PICO question (with PICo variant)

P	Patient, population or problem	
I	Intervention, prognostic factor or phenomenon of interest	
C	Comparison	Co = Context
O	Outcome	

 ## ACTIVITY 2.1 WRITING A PICO QUESTION

The question used for the research proposal may not be exactly the same as the question that is used to guide the literature search. Using the PICO mnemonic, take Natasha's working research question, and turn it into a searchable question for a literature review.

After you have placed the components of the search question under the PICO mnemonic, and you have looked at our suggested response on p. 40, consider what could be refined. For instance, while P representing primigravidae women may well be sufficient, if Natasha is interested in culture as a variable, she may want to focus this down by comparing white women from European Caucasian backgrounds with black women from Africa. By playing around with the mnemonic Natasha could add these terms into the PICO at P and C. The purpose of the PICO is simply a device to help you to refine your literature search question and hence your list of key terms. As mentioned, you could adapt the PICO to suit a qualitative study, designating 'Co' as 'context'.

CONSULT WITH YOUR RESEARCH LIBRARIAN

Once you have run your question through the PICO mnemonic, and have your list of key terms, visit your research librarian. Each database that you use to search will use slightly different subject headings and key terms as well as having the capacity for different search functions. For instance, Natasha and Liang will probably want to limit their searches in the first instance to studies published in the last 10 years. Liang may also want to limit his search to only previous studies that used an RCT (randomized controlled trial) design. A research librarian can help to set up the search strategy for this purpose.

TYPES OF LITERATURE

The literature for a review broadly falls into two kinds. The peer reviewed literature that includes refereed journal articles describing research studies, as well as theoretical arguments, is called the black literature. The non-peer reviewed literature that includes reports, books and theses is called the grey literature.

The black literature is the repository of scientific research papers, as the papers in this literature have been through various levels of peer review. The black literature on any topic should be relatively easy to find as almost all papers published in this literature are electronically indexed, which makes it possible to search for previous studies using the scientific bibliographic databases. Hence the black literature is the authoritative and accessible source of previous research. Reviewing this literature enables the current state of knowledge in the field to be established.

Not all information needed to justify a study will be contained in the black literature. For instance, background information about a problem (such as national disease rates) or the evaluation of a local intervention may only be written up in government or organizational reports. In many cases these reports are not peer reviewed. Also, this grey literature may not be indexed in the scientific bibliographic databases and therefore these reports can be difficult to identify. Hence, the grey literature can be the source of important information, but is not as authoritative or as accessible as the black literature. That said, information from reports from recognized government organizations and research institutes will most likely be of high quality, and access to these reports has been made much easier with the development of internet search engines.

Table 2.2   An example of methodologies in articles summarized by Natasha

Author/ date	Title	Aims/Objectives	Participants/ trimester	Research design	Findings
Goodman & Tyer-Viola, 2010	'Detection, Treatment, and Referral of Perinatal Depression and Anxiety by Obstetrical Providers'	To assess rates of detection, treatment, and referral of maternal depression and anxiety by obstetrical providers during pregnancy and 6 weeks post-partum.	Convenience sample ($n = 491$) screened for depression and anxiety during 3rd trimester and 6 weeks post-partum.	Questionnaires: Edinburgh Postnatal Depression Scale (EPDS) and patient Health Questionnaire. Data analysed using descriptive statistics.	23% of participants screened positive for an anxiety disorder or high levels of depressive symptoms or both prenatally; 17% positive at 6 weeks post-partum. Only 15% of positively screened participants had evidence of any mental health treatment in their electronic medical record during pregnancy.
Byrne et al., 2014	'Effectiveness of a mindfulness-based childbirth education pilot study on maternal self-efficacy and fear of childbirth (MBCE)'	To test the feasibility and effectiveness of using MBCE which aimed to reduce fear of birth, anxiety, and stress and improve maternal self-efficacy. Also to determine acceptability and feasibility of the MBCE protocol.	18 women (18–28 weeks gestation) completed intervention programme.	A single-arm pilot study of the MBCE intervention used a repeated-measures design. Programme ran weekly x 8 sessions.	Missing data allowed only 12 participants' data to be analysed. Statistically significant improvements and large effect size were observed for childbirth self-efficacy and fear of childbirth. Improvements in depression, mindfulness and birth outcome expectations were underpowered. Postnatally significant improvements were found in anxiety whereas improvements in mindfulness, stress, and fear of birth were significant at a less conservative alpha level.

(Continued)

Author/ date	Title	Aims/Objectives	Participants/ trimester	Research design	Findings
Ruiz-Robledillo et al, 2015	'Sleep during the third trimester of pregnancy: the role of depression and anxiety'	To analyse the effect of depression on sleep during the 3rd trimester controlling for anxiety.	143 women: depressed ($n = 77$) and non-depressed ($n = 66$).	Measures: EPDS; State Anxiety Inventory (STAI-S).	A marginally significant multivariate effect of anxiety was found for sleep. When controlling for anxiety, a significant multivariate effect of depression was found for sleep. Tests of between-subject effects, controlling for anxiety, revealed a significant univariate effect of depression on the number of awakenings during the night. When controlling for anxiety, depressed women revealed a higher number of awakenings and of hours spent trying to fall asleep.
Penacoba-Peunte et al, 2013	'Coping Strategies of Spanish pregnant women and their impact on anxiety and depression'	To analyse coping strategies in 1st trimester of low-risk pregnancies, their relationships to sociodemographic and pregnancy variables and their ability to predict anxiety and depression in the 3rd trimester.	Participants were 285 Spanish women in the 1st trimester, of whom 122 were followed into the 3rd trimester.	Coping strategies were measured with a self-reported inventory (Coping Strategies Questionnaire). For anxiety and depression, the Spanish version of the Symptom Check List 90-R was used. Sociodemographic and pregnancy data were collected with a questionnaire designed by the research team.	The use of problem-focused coping was stable; variations occurred in emotion-focused coping. Age, educational level, employment, planned pregnancy, previous childbirth and previous miscarriage were associated with adaptive coping. Coping strategies predicting anxiety and depressive symptoms were overt emotional expression and social support seeking. Coping through religion predicted anxiety.

MANAGING THE REVIEW

Two tips for managing a review of the literature are: first, use a software package such as Endnote, Reference Manager, Mendeley or Zotero to help you to conveniently store the citation details and summarize findings of articles. The second tip is to draw up a table of the retrieved studies as a way of comparing one study with others (see Table 2.2.). Table 2.2 shows an example of the methodologies of some studies Natasha reviewed. Additional columns could be added (e.g. ethnicity, nationality, age of participants, socio-economic background), depending upon your concepts of interest.

LOOKING FOR A GAP IN THE ANALYSED LITERATURE TO JUSTIFY A PROPOSAL

There are many guides for critically analysing the literature and you may like to consider the ones that we have used for qualitative studies and for quantitative studies. Critical review guidelines for qualitative studies and quantitative studies are included as Appendix A and Appendix B respectively at the end of this book (Schneider et al., 2016).

In this section we will cover some points that are relevant for a literature review suitable for a research proposal template that may only allow a few pages for this. A proposal literature review needs to be short, concise and sharp, compared to the literature review in a thesis that can be detailed and more expansive. A ball park figure for the number of studies reviewed for a proposal would be around 30 and so it is important to select the studies that best demonstrate the state of research knowledge in the selected field.

It is important to note similar concepts, how variables are defined, research approaches, samples and methods of data collection and analysis. Look also for consistency and differences in findings across studies, as well as the gaps: these should be made clear in the literature review.

ILLUSTRATION – LOOKING FOR A GAP

An example will illustrate this point. In reviewing studies on cognition in pregnancy for her PhD, one of the authors of this Guide (Schneider, 1989) analysed similar studies on the topic, cognition in pregnancy, to identify discrepancies. This enabled her to identify the methodological gap that her research could fill. Differences in the type and frequency of administration of psychological learning tests were obvious, however, the most distinguishing feature across all of the reviewed studies was the absence of baseline data. This was a serious omission because, without baseline data, there was no way of establishing how the women performed cognitively prior to becoming pregnant. While clinicians, and also the research studies, reported that unusually high levels of hormones adversely affected pregnant women cognitively, psychologically and physiologically, the extent to which this occurred remained unclear and uncertain in the absence of baseline data.

Draw conclusions and provide a judgement about the literature reviewed in order to support the reason for undertaking your research: that it is important and worth-while, and that the findings of your study will make a difference to the topic area investigated. Indicate precisely where your research question fits into the current and earlier literature. If little research has been conducted on your topic, it may be that you have to use any older or seminal literature available. Also, indicate how the design of your study will provide more information and enhance, enlarge, or extend the present knowledge base, that is, the contribution your study will make.

What follows are two examples of the literature search for the background and justification of Natasha's and Liang's studies.

READ–REFLECT–RESPOND 2.2

CRITIQUE OF NATASHA'S AND LIANG'S REVIEWS

Read Natasha's and Liang's literature reviews. Choose one to critique using the checklist below to identify the strengths and weaknesses of the review. Also, consider if the working title of their project accurately conveys the contents of the literature review. Do you think the review would persuade the committee of the relevance of the research project? Give reasons for your comments. On pp. 41–2 we have provided an example of how we have undertaken a critique of Liang's review.

CHECKLIST FOR A PROPOSAL LITERATURE REVIEW

1. Is the issue introduced and the impact and importance of the topic established?
2. Is the state of knowledge established about what is known and what is not known?
3. Are the study types described including the differences in design, sample, data collection and analysis as well as the method gaps?
4. Are the consistencies and differences in findings described as well as the content gaps?
5. Are the study concepts clearly defined?
6. Is the review of the literature sufficiently critical, that is, in examining the differences and similarities in the reviewed studies?
7. Is the literature review comprehensive, such as in using recent articles from refereed journals and in using primary sources?
8. Are only those studies relevant to building the case for the proposed study included in the review?
9. Is the justification for undertaking the proposed study convincing and clearly stated?
10. Has the researcher provided a convincing argument that the research will make a significant contribution to the body of knowledge that already exists on the topic?

BACKGROUND AND JUSTIFICATION FOR NATASHA'S STUDY

Natasha's working title is 'An investigation into pregnant women's experiences of ambivalence, anxiety and fears in the first trimester of pregnancy, and how they cope with their feelings.'

Background and justification

Pregnancy can be experienced as a period of physical, emotional and social upheaval (Ruiz-Robledillo et al., 2015; Schneider, 2002; Welldon, 1988). Anxiety in pregnancy has been referred to as 'a potential crisis state' (Gross and Pattison, 2007), and 10 to 20% of women suffer from mental health problems during pregnancy (Ayers and Shakespeare, 2015). High levels of stress and anxiety in pregnancy are known to have adverse effects on birth outcomes (Ding et al., 2014), such as a negative impact on fetal development (Kinsella and Monk, 2009), and increased rates of preterm delivery, reduced birthweight, and smaller head circumference (Lobel et al., 2008; Alderdice and Lynn, 2011). It is therefore important that a woman's emotional status be identified and addressed very early in pregnancy. It is equally important to understand how she copes with her emotions: this assessment could be done in the early weeks of her pregnancy. Once identified, appropriate and supportive social and educational interventions can be designed to alleviate the pernicious effects of stress and anxiety, to assist the woman to develop her coping strategies, and to enable her to enjoy a stable, happy pregnancy.

A woman's experience of pregnancy is influenced by psychological, biological and sociological events, interactions with important others in her life, health care professionals, education, the community in which she lives, and the kinds of information she receives or has access to. Studies investigating anxiety and fear in pregnancy have been conducted with women at various stages of pregnancy and the post-partum period, for instance exploring women's levels of childbirth fear in the third trimester (Goodman and Tyer-Viola, 2010; Hall et al., 2009, Ruiz-Robledillo et al., 2015), anxiety and depressive symptoms in the second and third trimesters (Bayrampour et al., 2015), comparing benefits of intervention on anxiety in the second trimester of pregnancy (Salehi et al., 2016), post-partum anxiety (Byrne et al., 2014; Lonstein, 2007), anxiety symptoms and coping strategies at various stages of pregnancy (George et al., 2013; Ip, Tang and Goggins 2009; Lee et al., 2007; McDonald et al., 2013; Witteveen, 2016), and unplanned pregnancy (Barton et al., 2017). However, there is no published study on how low-risk pregnant women perceive and cope with anxiety and fear in the first 12 weeks of gestation; a period compounded by extreme tiredness, potential ambivalence, and often nausea and vomiting.

Pregnancy is a time of dependence and vulnerability, and a pregnant woman, if she is having her baby in a hospital, becomes a patient, further increasing her perception of a dependent and subordinate role in the health care system. The stereotype that motherhood comes naturally to women may have no basis in fact but, nevertheless, may play an important part in her feelings, attitude, and experiences of pregnancy and, most importantly, her expectations of herself at this time. Feelings of anxiety and fear in the first trimester can lead to further stress for a woman who is trying to cope, especially if she is employed, with fatigue, ambivalence, morning sickness and vomiting.

The early weeks of pregnancy would be an appropriate time to introduce women, at their first antenatal visit, to maternal self-efficacy programmes. There is evidence to show that programmes focused on mental health reduce anxiety, depression and fear of childbirth (Bastani et al., 2005; Byrne et al., 2014; Ip Tang and Goggins, 2009). These types of programmes can be advertised in the clinic and women invited to participate in the early weeks of their pregnancy. It would also be evidence of a researcher using evidence-based best practice.

The aim of the study is to identify situations and events which cause anxiety and fear in the first trimester of pregnancy; the objective is to discover and analyse women's perceptions of their anxiety and fear through the administration of a questionnaire and one in-depth interview during the last days of the first trimester. Unless recognized and addressed, feelings of anxiety and fear can persist throughout pregnancy and cloud an event which should be a happy and healthy time. A grounded theory 'emic' approach using in-depth interviews will be used in order to understand the perceptions, experiences, feelings, and behaviours of the women. The information provided by the women will guide health professionals in designing a psycho-educational intervention programme to assist women to cope.

BACKGROUND AND JUSTIFICATION FOR LIANG'S STUDY

NOTE : For critique on how up to date the publications are, it should be noted that this work was written in 2006.

Liang's working question is, 'Can a system of chronic disease care planning be implemented in General Practice that leads to positive client outcomes? Would the system be feasible within the role and skill capacity of nurses working in General Practice and within the current levels of funding available for General Practice services?'

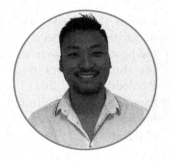

Background and justification

As in many other countries, depression, diabetes and heart disease represent three of the leading disease burdens in Australia with all three conditions being identified as

National Health Priority Areas (National Health Priority Action Council, 2006). Coronary heart disease and diabetes frequently co-exist and the impact of depression on both conditions has been shown to significantly adversely impact on mortality and morbidity outcomes (Ali et al., 2006; Egede et al., 2005). These chronic conditions are managed in the main in General Practice, and it is in this setting where the majority of patients seek help. The management of these conditions in rural areas, where there is a lack of access to specialist referral services, represents an additional challenge.

The international literature has shown that chronic illness care benefits from comprehensive and multifaceted health service delivery, and that General Practices are central to the success of coordinated chronic disease management (CDM) (Lewis and Dixon, 2004; Wagner, 2004). GPs often have limited time to manage the complex care needs of their patients and could benefit from additional resources to help in CDM.

In Australia the system of chronic disease care has been strengthened with the provision of new funding, and there has been initially slow but steady uptake of the new funding item numbers for chronic disease, especially those for mental health (McDonald et al., 2006). The Medicare Benefits Schedule (MBS) chronic disease management item numbers, introduced in July 2005, offer a potential solution but it requires changes in practice organization as outlined here.

This proposal, which has been developed with advice from GPs and leaders from divisions of General Practice, will demonstrate how chronic diseases can be better managed using the item numbers. The study will also test a workforce solution by increasing the skills of practice nurses to manage heart disease, diabetes, and depression related disorders. This study will not add to the work of GPs nor will it reduce their income. It will improve outcomes for patients while using existing sources of funding, particularly the new item numbers.

This project will develop, test and implement a model for assessment and treatment that is based both on sound research findings and the way that Australian General Practice is developing the care of chronic illness. Programmes like *More Allied Health Services* (Department of Health, undated(a)) and *Better Access to Psychiatrists, Psychologists and General Practitioners through the MBS (Better Access) Initiative* (Department of Health, undated(b)) provide opportunities for GPs to be better trained, and to make referrals to these services. This project, which is aligned with the consultation draft of the National Chronic Disease Strategy, the National Service Improvement Framework for Diabetes, and the National Service Improvement Framework for Heart, Stroke and Vascular Disease, will also train the extended team, within and outside the General Practice, to manage an integrated shared care model which can be sustained under the MBS CDM items introduced in July 2005. Our approach uses the world's best model for delivery of CDM including evidence-based guidelines and interprofessional teamwork in General Practice (Davis, Wagner and Groves, 2000; Dixon et al., 2004; Groves and Wagner, 2005; Hunkeler et al., 2006; Katon, 2000; Raftery et al., 2005; Simon, 2006; Wagner, 2001; Wagner and Groves, 2002; Wagner and Simon, 2001).

A 'Collaborative Practice' is defined as 'groups of people who share a concern, a common set of problems, or a passion about a topic and who deepen their knowledge and expertise in this area by interacting on an ongoing basis' (Wenger et al., 2000). Communities of Practice, like Collaboratives, are internationally recognized ways of getting evidence into practice (Wenger et al., 2000). Both approaches are used in Australia by the National Institute of Clinical Studies and we are currently using this approach to improve the system of care for people with co-morbid depression and heart disease and/or diabetes to demonstrate best practice (National Institute of Clinical Studies, 2004a, 2004b).

Using a 'Collaborative Practice', this implementation study builds on evidence-based CDM models in General Practice that have largely been applied overseas to a single condition. We will demonstrate a best-practice model for the management of diabetes, heart disease and co-morbid depression in 20 General Practices in both urban and rural areas of Australia.

CONCLUSION

In this chapter we have covered the second step, the background and justification, in the development of a research proposal. Completion of this step means that you will have explained in your proposal that a study is needed because a problem exists for which further research is required. In providing this justification you will have identified a gap in our understanding of this problem, about which your proposed study will provide some answers. This is called filling the topic gap.

Your topic gap can be described within a theoretical or conceptual framework and the advantage of doing this is that the framework will help you to develop a list of possible study concepts and the relationship between them.

The study justification and conceptual framing occurs through the conduct of a critical and succinct literature review.

Having justified that a study is needed and by describing a gap in the literature, you are ready to write a research question as the final task in Step Two. The next step, Step Three, is about designing an appropriate study (research design) that can generate the data and analysis to fill the knowledge gap. Before moving onto this step, your final activity is to now complete Step Two on your own study, that is, to describe the background, to argue that a study is justified, and to write a working study title.

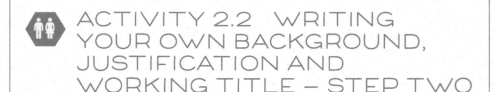

ACTIVITY 2.2 WRITING YOUR OWN BACKGROUND, JUSTIFICATION AND WORKING TITLE – STEP TWO

Having critiqued the literature review of either Natasha or Liang, now it is time to conduct your own review as a way of providing the background and justification for your study and to write a working title. This is the second step in developing a research proposal and to do this you should complete the following activities.

1.   Use the PICO mnemonic to write a literature search question.
2.   Consult your research librarian to list your search key terms and to establish the search strategy for the databases that you will search on.
3.   Run the search and retrieve the relevant studies.

4. Draw up a table of these studies.
5. Write the proposal background and justification of about two pages.
6. Devise a working title for your study.
7. Use the checklist on p. 32 to ensure that you have covered the essential points.

REVISION

Below you will find five statements related to the content of this chapter. Indicate whether you believe each statement to be true or false. The answers are given on p. 43.

1. The importance of a problem can be determined by looking at the extent of the problem (how large it is) as well as the impact on those who are affected.

   T/F

2. Every research project should be guided by a theoretical framework.

   T/F

3. It is NOT necessary to conduct a literature review if it is obvious that there is either a topic or a method gap.

   T/F

4. Another term for the background and justification of a study is the significance of a study.

   T/F

5. In most research it is helpful to operationally define the concepts to be investigated before the study commences.

   T/F

REFERENCES

Alderdice, F. and Lynn, F. (2011) Factor structure of the prenatal distress questionnaire. *Midwifery,* 27(4): 553–559

Ali, S., Stone, M., Peters, J., Davies, M.J. and Khunti, K. (2006) The prevalence of co-morbid depression in adults with Type 2 diabetes: a systematic review and meta-analysis. *Diabetic Medicine,* 23(11): 1165–1173.

Ayers, S. and Shakespeare, J. (2015) Should perinatal mental health be everyone's business? *Primary Health Care Research & Development,* 16(4): 323–325.

Barton, K., Redshaw, M., Quigley, M.A. and Caron, C. (2017) Unplanned pregnancy and subsequent psychological distress in partnered women: a cross-sectional study of the role of relationship quality and wider social support. *BMC Pregnancy and Childbirth,* 17: 44.

Bastani, F., Hidarnia, A., Kazemnejad, A., Vafaei, M. and Kashanian, M. (2005) A randomized controlled trial of the effects of applied relaxation training on reducing anxiety and perceived stress in pregnant women. *Journal of Midwifery & Women's Health,* 50(4): e36–40.

Bayrampour, H., McDonald, S. and Tough, S. (2015) Risk factors of transient and persistent anxiety during pregnancy. *Midwifery,* 31(6): 582–589.

Byrne, J., Hauck, Y., Fisher, C., Bayes, S. and Schutze, R. (2014) Effectiveness of a mindfulness-based childbirth education pilot study on maternal self-efficacy and fear of childbirth. *Journal of Midwifery & Women's Health,* 59(2): 192–197.

Davis, R.M., Wagner, E.G. and Groves, T. (2000) Advances in managing chronic disease. *BMJ,* 320: 525–526.

Department of Health (undated(a)) 8.2. Allied health workforce. (www.health. gov.au/internet/publications/publishing.nsf/Content/work-review-australian-government-health-workforce-programs-toc~chapter-8-developing-dental-allied-health-workforce~chapter-8-allied-health-workforce). [Last acccesed 5 September 2017]

Department of Health (undated(b)) Better Access to Psychiatrists, Psychologists and General Practitioners through the MBS (Better Access) initiative (www.health. gov.au/mentalhealth-betteraccess). [last accessed 5 September 2017]

Ding, X.X., Wu, Y.L., Xu, S.J., Zhu, R.P., Jia, X.M., Zhang, S.F., Huang, K., Zhu, P., Hao, J.H. and Tao, F.B. (2014) Maternal anxiety during pregnancy and adverse birth outcomes: a systematic review and meta-analysis of prospective cohort studies. *Journal of Affective Disorders,* 159: 103–110.

Dixon, J., Lewis, R., Rosen, R., Finlayson, B. and Gray, D. (2004) Can the NHS learn from US managed care organizations? *BMJ,* 328(7433): 223–225.

Egede, L., Nietert, P. and Zeng, D. (2005) Depression and all-cause and coronary heart disease mortality among adults with and without diabetes. *Diabetes Care,* 28(6): 1339–1345.

George, A., Luz, R.F., De Tychey, C., Thilly, N., and Spitz, E. (2013) Anxiety symptoms and coping strategies in the perinatal period. *BMC Pregnancy and Childbirth,* 13: 233.

Goodman, J.H. and Tyer-Viola, L. (2010) Detection, treatment, and referral of perinatal depression and anxiety by obstetrical providers. *Journal of Women's Health,* 19(3): 477–490.

Gray, K. and Sockolow, P.S. (2016) Conceptual models in health informatics research: a literature review and suggestions for development. *JMIR Medical Informatics,* 4(1): e7.

Gross, H. and Pattison, H. (2007) *Sanctioning Pregnancy. A Psychological Perspective on the Paradoxes and Culture of Research.* London: Routledge.

Groves, T. and Wagner, E.H. (2005) High quality care for people with chronic diseases. *BMJ,* 330: 609–610.

Hall, W.A., Hauck, Y.L., Carty, E.M., Hutton, E.K., Fenwick, J. and Stoll, K. (2009) Childbirth fear, anxiety, fatigue, and sleep deprivation in pregnant women. *Journal of Obstetric, Gynecologic & Neonatal Nursing,* 38(5): 567–576.

Harrison, S. and Gibbons, C. (2013) Nursing student perceptions of concept maps: from theory to practice. *Nursing Education Perspectives,* 34(6): 395–399.

Hunkeler, E.M., Katon, W., Tang, L., Williams, J.W., Kroenke, K., Lin, E.H.B., Harpole, L.H., Arean, P., Levine, S., Grypma, L.M., Hargreaves, W.A. and

Unutzer, J. (2006) Long term outcomes from the IMPACT randomised trial for depressed elderly patients in primary care. *BMJ*, 332: 259–263.

Ip, W-Y., Tang, C.S.K. and Goggins, W.B. (2009) An educational intervention to improve women's ability to cope with childbirth. *Journal of Clinical Nursing*, 18(15): 2125–2135.

Israeloff, R. (1985) *Coming to Terms*. New York: Penguin.

Joanna Briggs Institute (2014) *Reviewers' Manual*. University of Adelaide. (https://joannabriggs.org/assets/docs/sumari/ReviewersManual-2014.pdf). [last accessed 5 September 2017]

Katon, W. (2000) Improvement of outcomes in chronic illness. *Archives of Family Medicine*, 9: 709–711.

Kinsella, M.T. and Monk, C. (2009) Impact of maternal stress, depression and anxiety on fetal neurobehavioral development. *Clinical Obstetrics and Gynecology*, 52(3): 425–440.

Lee, A.M., Lam, S.K., Sze Mun Lau, S.M., Chong C.S.Y., Chui, H.W. and Fong, D.Y.T. (2007) Prevalence, course and risk factors for antenatal anxiety and depression. *Obstetrics & Gynecology*, 110(5): 1102–1112.

Lewis, R. and Dixon, J. (2004) Rethinking management of chronic diseases. *BMJ*, 328: 220–222.

Lobel, M., Cannella, L.D., Graham, E.J., Devincent, J.C., Schneider, J. and Meyer, A.B. (2008) Pregnancy-specific stress, prenatal health behaviours and birth outcomes. *Health Psychology*, 27(5): 604–615.

Lonstein, J.S. (2007) Regulation of anxiety during the postpartum period. *Frontiers in Neuroendocrinology*, 28(2–3): 115–41.

McDonald, J., Cumming, J., Harris, M., Powell-Davies, G. and Burns, P. (2006) *Systematic review of comprehensive primary care models*. Canberra: Australian Primary Health Care Research Institute.

McDonald, S.W., Lyon, A.W., Benzies, K.M., McNeil, D.A., Lye, S.J., Dolan, S.M., Pennell, C.E., Bocking, A.D. and Tough, S.C. (2013) The All our Babies pregnancy cohort: design, methods and participant characteristics. *BMC Pregnancy and Childbirth*, 13 (Suppl.1):S2.

National Health Priority Action Council (2006) *National Chronic Disease Strategy and the Frameworks*. Canberra, Australia: Department of Health and Ageing.

National Institute of Clinical Studies (2004a) *National Emergency Department Collaborative Report*. Melbourne: NICS.

National Institute of Clinical Studies (2004b) Emergency Care Community of Practice Program. *Developing Communities of Practice and how they apply to the health context*. Melbourne: NICS.

Penacoba-Peunte, C., Carmona-Monge, F.J., Marin-Morales, D. and Naber, K. (2013) 'Coping strategies of Spanish pregnant women and their impact on anxiety and depression', *Research in Nursing and Health*, 36(1): 54–64.

Plumb, M. and Kautz (2014) 'Innovation within an Early Childhood Education and Care Organisation: A Tri-Perspective Analysis of the Appropriation of IT', 25th Australasian Conference on Information Systems, 8–10 December, Auckland, New Zealand.

Raftery, J.P, Yao, G.L., Murchie, P., Campbell, N.C. and Ritchie, L.D. (2005) Cost effectiveness of nurse led secondary prevention clinics for coronary heart disease in primary care: follow up of a randomised controlled trial. *BMJ,* 330(7493): 707.

Raibley, J.R. (2012) Happiness is not well-Being. *Journal of Happiness Studies,* 13(6): 1105–1129.

Ruiz-Robledillo, N., Canario, C., Dias, C.C., Moya-Albiol, L. and Figueriredo, B. (2015) Sleep during the third trimester of pregnancy: the role of depression and anxiety. *Psychology, Health & Medicine,* 20(8): 1–6.

Salehi, F., Pourasghar, M., Khalilian, A. and Shahhosseini, Z. (2016) Comparison of group cognitive behavioural therapy and interactive lectures in reducing anxiety during pregnancy. *Medicine,* 95(43): e5224.

Schneider, Z. (1989) *Thinking and Learning in Pregnancy.* Doctoral thesis. Monash University, Australia.

Schneider, Z. (2002) An Australian study of women's experiences of their first pregnancy. *Midwifery,* 18(3): 238–249.

Schneider, Z., Whitehead, D., LoBiondo-Wood, G. and Haber, J. (2016) *Nursing and Midwifery Research: methods and appraisal for evidence-based practice* 5th edn. Austrialia: Elsevier.

Sercekus, P. and Mete, S. (2010) Effects of antenatal education on maternal prenatal and postpartum adaptation. *Journal of Advanced Nursing,* 66(5): 999–1010.

Simon, G. (2006) Collaborative care for depression. *BMJ,* 332: 249–250.

Wagner, E.H. (2001) Meeting the needs of chronically ill people. *BMJ,* 323: 945–946.

Wagner, E.H. (2004) Chronic Disease Care. *BMJ,* 328: 177–178.

Wagner, E.H. and Groves, T. (2002) Care for chronic diseases. *BMJ,* 325: 913–914.

Wagner, E.H. and Simon, G.E. (2001) Managing depression in primary care. *BMJ,* 322: 746–747.

Welldon, E.V. (1988) *Mother Madonna Whore. The Idealization and Denigration of Motherhood.* London: The Guilford Press.

Wenger, E., McDermott, R. and Snyder, W.M. (2000) *Cultivating Communities of Practice.* Boston: Harvard Business School Press.

Witteveen, A.B., De Cock, P., Muizink, A.C., De Jonge, A., Klomp, T., Westemeng, M. and Geerte, C.C. (2016) Pregnancy related anxiety and general anxious or depressed mood and the choice for birth setting: a secondary data-analysis of the DELIVER study. *BMC Pregnancy and Childbirth,* 16(1): 363.

ANSWERS TO ACTIVITIES

ACTIVITY 2.1

SUGGESTED ANSWER

P　　= primigravidae

I　　= anxiety, locus of control, coping strategy

Co　= first trimester of pregnancy

READ-REFLECT-RESPOND 2.2 USING THE CHECKLIST TO CRITIQUE LIANG'S REVIEW

Example critique of the background and justification of Liang's review against the checklist

1.	Is the issue introduced and the impact and importance of the topic established?	Yes – paragraph one and paragraph three sentence one cover this.
		'As in many other countries, depression, diabetes and heart disease represent three of the leading disease burdens in Australia with all three conditions being identified as National Health Priority Areas … The management of these conditions in rural areas, where there is a lack of access to specialist referral services, represents an additional challenge … In Australia the system of chronic disease care has been strengthened with the provision of new funding, and there has been initially slow but steady uptake of the new funding item numbers for chronic disease, especially those for mental health.'
2.	Is the state of knowledge established about what is known and what is not known?	Yes – paragraph two sentence one covers this.
		'The international literature has shown that chronic illness care benefits from comprehensive and multifaceted health service delivery, and that General Practices are central to the success of coordinated chronic disease management.'
3.	Are the study types described including the differences in design, sample, data collection and analysis including the method gaps?	No.
4.	Are the consistencies and differences in findings described as well as the content gaps?	Not consistencies and differences – but gap is identified in paragraph seven.
		'Using a "Collaborative Practice", this implementation study builds on evidence-based CDM models in General Practice that have largely been applied overseas to a single condition. We will demonstrate a best-practice model for the management of diabetes, heart disease and co-morbid depression in 20 General Practices in both urban and rural areas of Australia.'

(Continued)

5.	Are the studied concepts clearly defined?	Yes – paragraph six covers this. 'A "Collaborative Practice" is defined as "groups of people who share a concern, a common set of problems, or a passion about a topic and who deepen their knowledge and expertise in this area by interacting on an ongoing basis"… Both approaches are used in Australia by the National Institute of Clinical Studies and we are currently using this approach to improve the system of care for people with co-morbid depression and heart disease and/or diabetes to demonstrate best practice.'
6.	Is the review of the literature sufficiently critical, that is, in examining the differences and similarities in the reviewed studies?	No.
7.	Is the literature review comprehensive, such as in using recent articles from refereed journals and in using primary sources?	Yes.
8.	Are only those studies that are relevant to building the case for the proposed study included in the review?	Yes.
9.	Is the justification for undertaking the proposed study convincing and clearly stated?	Yes – paragraph two and seven refer to the literature. The justification, based on the study advancing previous research and hence filling a research gap, is referred to in paragraph six. Previous research focused on single disease compared to this proposed study on co-morbidity.
10.	Has the researcher provided a convincing argument that the research will make a significant contribution to the body of knowledge that already exists on the topic?	Yes – paragraph seven covers this. Using a 'Collaborative Practice', this implementation study builds on evidence-based CDM models in General Gractice that have largely been applied overseas to a single condition. We will demonstrate a best-practice model for the management of diabetes, heart disease and co-morbid depression in 20 General Practices in both urban and rural areas of Australia.

REVISION STATEMENTS

1. T
2. F
3. F
4. F
5. T

You can find Appendix A on Critical review guidelines for qualitative studies and Appendix B on Critical review guidelines for quantitative studies at the end of this book.

STEP THREE
RESEARCH APPROACH AND DESIGN

CONTENT

- Establishing the research question
- Choosing a research approach
- Justification of the research approach and methods
- Defining and operationalizing concepts for data collection
- The 'nuts and bolts' – sampling strategies/data collection/data analysis/limitations/demonstrating rigour

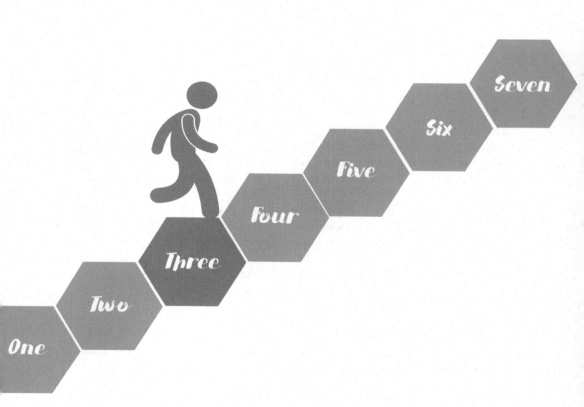

KEY TERMS/CONCEPTS

- Researchable question
- Rich data
- Thick description
- Three qualitative designs (phenomenology, ethnography and grounded theory)
- Two main quantitative designs – experimental and observational designs
- Causal association
- The 'so what?' question
- Operationalization of study concepts
- Rigour

INTRODUCTION

This chapter covers Step Three in a research proposal and deals with the research approach and design. This is the most important section of a research proposal. It is in this step that you describe the scientific methodology (research design) that guides the study. In this section of the proposal you need to show how all aspects of your study fit together into a coherent and logical research design that will answer the research question. While the success of a research proposal depends on all of the steps, regardless of how well all of the other steps are completed, if this third step is not clear and logical then the proposal will most likely be rejected. This is the 'engine room' of your research proposal.

ESTABLISHING THE RESEARCH QUESTION

The key starting point for the research design step is to establish a researchable question. You then ensure that the overall conceptual framework, the research paradigm and the pragmatic 'nuts and bolts' activities such as sampling, data collection and analysis are all appropriate to answer the question. Biddix (2009) states:

A research question is the fundamental core of a research project, study or review of literature. It focuses the study, determines the methodology, and guides all stages of inquiry, analysis, and reporting.

A good research question will facilitate the following processes:

- guide the research process;
- devise efficient literature search strategies;
- write a literature review;
- plan thesis chapters;
- construct a logical argument.

A good research question is one that achieves the following (Duke University, undated; Queensland University of Technology, undated):

- asks about something that is important;
- enables collection of data that can sustain an illuminating argument (rather than a yes/no response);
- is not too broad or narrow for a study within the available time and resources.

For example, the following is a poor research question, because it is too broad and requires a moral or ethical response to do with standards of practice rather than a research response.

Should health care workers convey a caring attitude towards clients?

Dealing with the same problem, the following research question: 'What do mental health workers consider to be appropriate behaviours in their practice to convey a caring attitude to adolescent clients of the opposite gender?' is a much better research question because it does the following:

- names the concepts to be studied, including the participants and setting;
- enables generation of data to build an argument related to these concepts;
- names the source and type of data to be collected.

READ-REFLECT-RESPOND 3.1
YOUR WORKING RESEARCH QUESTION

The working research question will usually be written at the end of the literature review or the start of the research design section.

We can ascertain Natasha's and Liang's research questions from the previous chapter.

Natasha's research question is:

What are pregnant women's experiences of ambivalence, anxiety and fear in the first trimester of pregnancy, and how do they cope with their feelings?

Liang's research question is:

Can a system of chronic disease care planning be implemented in General Practice that leads to positive client outcomes? Would the system be feasible within the role and skill capacity of nurses working in General Practice and within the current levels of funding available for General Practice services?

Do you think that these questions could be improved? See our suggested answer on p. 74.
Now draw on your response to Activity 2.2 (see p. 36) to write your own research question.

CHOOSING A RESEARCH APPROACH

Having established a working research question, the next part of Step Three is to decide which research approach will best answer the research question: a qualitative, quantitative or mixed methods approach. Right from the outset, decisions about the approach and then the specific design are important insofar as these must achieve the following:

- logically follow from the research question;
- best answer the research question;
- show how answering this research question using this approach will add to the current state of knowledge on a topic.

While this Guide is not a research text book on the differences between approaches and specific study designs, it is timely to provide an overview of major qualitative, quantitative and mixed methods designs, as each serves a different purpose and so needs a different decision-making logic and rationale to justify its use in a proposal. A qualitative approach aims to generate textual data to describe a phenomenon; a quantitative approach aims to generate numerical data to measure a phenomenon; a mixed methods paradigm seeks to do both.

The major difference between qualitative and quantitative research approaches, apart from the philosophical stance and conceptual underpinnings, is one of intention or purpose. An example of phenomenological qualitative research will illustrate this, particularly how this influences the logic for data collection and analysis.

In phenomenological qualitative research, the approach is to provide the opportunity for interviewees to think about, reflect on, explore, and examine a particular question (phenomenon) in relation to themselves, what meaning it has for them, and how they interpret their experience of it. This approach invites personal reflection about thoughts, feelings, and experiences. The interview is labelled 'in-depth' which implies a personal, searching, and detailed response and thus facilitates obtaining 'thick' description and 'rich' data. Taylor and Bogdan (1984: 77) define in-depth interviews as 'repeated face-to-face encounters between the researcher and informants directed toward understanding informants' perspectives on their lives, experiences or situations as expressed in their own words'. The terms 'rich' and 'thick' description also need definition. 'Rich' data are full and comprehensive accounts. 'Thick' description refers to 'capturing and conveying the full picture of behaviour being studied – holistically, comprehensively and in context' (Punch, 2006: 157). In phenomenological research, therefore, the intention is to obtain information, either verbally or in writing, from the unique perspective of the interviewee. The question of generalizability in qualitative research is not a key consideration and the number of study participants is usually not large. What is of relevance in phenomenological research is that the information obtained from participants is uniquely theirs. This is not to imply that there cannot be overlap with other participants' experiences. While the philosophy and concepts underpinning the major research approaches differ, they are united in their aim: the production of new information and hence new understandings.

READ–REFLECT–RESPOND 3.2
IN–DEPTH INTERVIEW

Read the following excerpts by women in their first trimester of pregnancy. Think of the definition of an in-depth interview. Would you consider the information in the following excerpts to be 'in-depth'? Give reasons for your answer.

1. '... and the tiredness, I wish someone had said: "You're going to be flattened". I felt angry that I hadn't been told. I felt so naive, a bit like a child phoning my mother and asking her how it would continue and what it all meant.'
2. 'I've felt very, very tired, and a bit down and imagining that I would never have the energy again to be any good – I think of myself as being strong and in control but now I feel that I'm not dealing with this and I'm losing confidence in myself.'

An overview of these major research approaches will alert you, while creating your own proposal, to the various nuances of meaning when considering design, data collection and data analysis.

QUALITATIVE APPROACHES

There are many different qualitative research approaches known as postpositivism (also called postempiricism) or interpretivism. Three major research approaches – phenomenology, ethnography and grounded theory – have differences in terms of design features around data collection and analysis. These will be briefly discussed.

Phenomenology

Phenomenological research is an inductive and descriptive research approach which aims to provide the opportunity for an individual to express their perceptions, interpretations and the meaning of an event from their perspective. In other words, the research approach is to seek self-expression from an insider's perspective, and how an individual constructs meaning of 'lived experience'. Van Manen (1990) identifies four distinct features of 'lived experience': lived space (spatiality); lived body (corporeality); lived time (temporality); and lived human relations (relationality). Data collection strategies in phenomenology include in-depth interviews, diaries, telephone conversations, observation, and written or oral self-reports.

Let us take as an example the cultural beliefs and attitudes towards pain of both patients and team members in a multicultural society. The pertinence of using a phenomenological approach becomes clear when considering the challenges facing a multicultural foreign and local health care team. The unique experiences and interpretations of pain, not only of the culturally diverse patients, but also the culturally diverse care team, must be acknowledged and respected throughout the research process. An example from a research study will illustrate how one phenomenological hermeneutical design was used. Winger et al. (2013) explored the experience of being an adolescent with chronic fatigue syndrome. Six boys and 12 girls, aged 12–18, were interviewed and asked for their personal experiences of living with the condition. The life-world experiences of the participants were analysed using a phenomenological hermeneutical approach (hermeneutics interpreted the text, while phenomenology aimed to understand the experiences). Data were analysed using three methodological steps: naive reading, thematic structural analysis and comprehensive understanding. The core theme 'sometimes it feels as if the world goes on without me' encompasses how the adolescents perceived their existence.

Ethnography

Ethnography is a qualitative social research method concerned with the study of cultures in natural settings, and aims to understand and elucidate a group's behaviour through the medium of their own culture. Researchers enter a research site and immerse themselves in the lives and culture of the group.

A central tenet of the ethnographic viewpoint is that a group's experiences are socially organized and the researcher is required to enter the research site. The researcher aims to learn about the group through the prism of its culture, and may incorporate aspects of gender, ethnicity, nationality, or whatever else the researcher considers relevant. Goodson and Vassar (2011: 4) suggest that the requirement to enter the site or the world of the group 'allows the researcher to take advantage of relative immersion in order to obtain thick descriptions'. In health care research the interest may be in some topic like type 1 diabetes or HIV and how the culture of a group influences a person's response to a diagnosis and subsequent disease management.

Pope (2005) relates her personal experience of conducting ethnographic research in a medical environment. Pope describes how she negotiated access and consent from the medical staff she observed in three separate studies involving anaesthetists and surgeons in the UK and the USA. She says: 'Ethnography is rooted in writing. Lengthy periods of observation require hours of copious note taking and writing' (Pope, 2005: 1182). Initially an outsider and a complete observer, she gradually became more integrated into the group.

Grounded theory

Unlike phenomenology and ethnography, grounded theory is not concerned so much with the data collection perspective (such as lived experience or cultural influence), but rather an approach to the analysis where the findings from the data are used to construct a framework or theory about the phenomenon/phenomena. Hence analysis is used to develop theory (or at least part of it), whereas phenomenological and ethnographic data collection and analysis are informed by, and add to, existing theory. The classic grounded theory approach enunciated by Glaser and Strauss (1967) has undergone adaptation and change, and the four proponents of grounded theory, Glaser, Strauss, Corbin and Charmaz, have proposed different versions of this approach. Data for grounded theory can come from interviews, observations, video tapes, and field notes.

A team of researchers (Sbaraini et al., 2011) used grounded theory methodology in their aim to provide a model for dental practice. They acknowledge the diversity of grounded theory methodology and suggest that, while many authors label their research grounded theory, they do not follow the basics of the methodology. The authors describe the fundamental components as openness, analysing immediately, coding and comparing, memo writing, theoretical sampling and theoretical saturation, and finally the production of a substantive theory. They stated that they 'developed a detailed model of the process of adapting preventive protocols into dental practice, and to analyse variation in this process in different dental practices' (Sbaraini et al., 2011: 136).

Table 3.1   Comparison of approaches to data analysis of popular qualitative methodologies

Research approach	Research focus	Type of data	Analysis strategies
Grounded theory	Human action and interaction	Anything relevant to the study can be data: • Interviews • Observations • Field notes	Coding (open, axial, selective) • Categorisation • Constant comparison
Phenomenology	The experience and meaning of phenomena	Texts, e.g. interview transcripts	Coding • Categorisation • Thematising • Interpreting
Ethnography	The social organization of experience	Anything relevant to the study can be data: • Interviews • Observations • Field notes	Coding • Categorising • Interpreting
Narrative	How individuals construct understanding of an event	Individuals' stories (usually interviews)	Coding • Thematising • Restorying
Descriptive exploratory	Explanation of phenomena	Anything relevant to the study can be data: • Interviews • Observations • Objects and artefacts • Documents	Coding • Content analysis • Summarizing

Source: Schneider et al., (2016) *Nursing and Midwifery Research: methods and appraisal for evidence-based practice* 5th edn. Australia: Elsevier. Reproduced with permission.

QUANTITATIVE APPROACHES

In natural sciences and social sciences, quantitative research is the investigation of observable phenomena using measurement tools and methods. Quantitative research comprises two main types of study design; observational design and experimental design (Shields and Smyth, 2016). Both designs have a similar purpose, which is through measurement to show the probable causal association between two or more variables, that is, that one variable (predictor) is the likely cause of the other variable (outcome). Both design types seek the following:

- objectivity through valid and accurate instruments;
- generalizability of findings beyond study participants through probability sampling techniques;
- freedom from the influence of extraneous non-study-related variables through control of these variables.

The emphasis is on generalizing the findings obtained from the study sample in such a way that the researcher is able to infer, on the basis of probability, that these findings would apply to the larger population of the same participant types. Quantitative studies seek to answer questions like 'is a diabetes discharge management programme effective in reducing hospital readmission?' and 'investigating the extent and causes of perforations in surgical gloves', and 'what factors enhance and impede adult Chinese migrants' learning of English as a second language?' At first glance, the last question may not appear to lend itself to straightforward quantification of responses; in such cases research instruments and questionnaires are designed to produce data in numerical form (see Gillespie and Chaboyer, 2016).

Observational designs

The aim of observational designs is to observe and identify variables of interest and examine the relationship between those variables. Subtypes of observational designs are descriptive, correlational, cross-sectional, retrospective, case-control, cohort and longitudinal. In many instances it is either not possible or ethical to conduct an experimental study, which is discussed below. For instance it would be unethical to conduct an experiment on the causal association between a high fat diet and the development of obesity. It would not be ethical to intentionally give one group an intervention (high fat diet) that we think might be the cause of harm (obesity). For these problems it is possible, however, to conduct observational studies of phenomena in the natural world to see if one variable (high fat diet) is associated with another variable (obesity) and then, depending on the type of observational design, to draw inferences about whether this association is likely to be causal. A study where the measurement is cross sectional and only conducted once leads to a weak level of evidence about the causal association. For example, just because we find in a study sample that people who eat a high fat are more obese compared to those who do not eat a high fat diet, we cannot draw a causal inference that one leads to the other. We do not know which variable came first, and so it could even be that people who are obese (for whatever reason) are attracted to a high fat diet. If we conducted an observational study with longitudinal repeated measurements across two groups, such as a cohort or case-control design, it would be possible to make more confident inferences that one variable leads to another. This is because the design separates the sample into two groups and follows each group either forward (cohort) or back into their history (case-control) to see if exposure to one variable precedes the development of the other variable.

An example of an observational study was by Mjaaland et al. (2011) who video-taped, using a still camera and microphones, 96 medical consultations. The VR-CoDES (Verona coding Definitions of Emotional Sequences) were used to code the patients' negative emotional cues and concerns (NECC). Descriptive statistics were used for analysis with the z test to compare proportions between groups. While NECC were observed in more than half of the consultations (109 negative emotional cues and 54 concerns) more than half of the concerns were not preceded by these cues. There were no significant differences found related to the gender or age of patients or physician, or the specialty of the physician. The purpose was to better understand the detection of patients' emotional distress by health providers. The implications derived from this study are that patients' expressions of emotional issues are subtle and physicians should be trained to identify and respond to them.

Experimental designs

In experimental designs the researcher seeks to manipulate the predictor variable (for example, a specific intervention such as an exercise programme prior to hospital discharge), to see if the outcome is different for those receiving the intervention compared with those who do not receive it (control or comparison group). The researcher seeks to control the study so that ideally the participants in both groups are similar and that the settings from which the data are collected are similar. This enables the researcher to conclude that any difference in outcome between the two groups is due to the intervention. Hence, experimental studies provide the highest level of evidence that a predictor variable (such as level of exercise) is the cause of an outcome variable (such as level of obesity). The main type of experimental design is the randomized controlled trial or RCT. However, where some level of control is not possible (for instance, the researcher manipulates the intervention but control and randomisation are lacking), an intervention study would be called a quasi-experimental design.

There is a very large variety of experimental designs, and we have elected to provide an example of a randomized controlled trial (RCT). The RCT by Laffin et al. (2015) compared the effectiveness of two creams in minimizing the incidence of moist desquamation in a tropical setting and which was most acceptable to patients receiving radiation therapy. Participants ($n = 255$) were stratified according to breast or chest wall radiation treatment and randomly assigned to a group using a moisturizing cream or barrier cream. Radiation skin reactions were assessed weekly and patients were telephoned one month post treatment for a final skin assessment. At completion of treatment 15% of participants had moist desquamation. An additional 26% self-reported this at follow-up. The barrier cream significantly reduced the incidence of moist desquamation during radiation treatment to the chest wall.

Table 3.2   Continuum of quantitative research designs

Design increasing control and ability to assign causality	Subtypes	Features
Observational	Descriptive	Describes variables
	Correlational	Examines relationships between variables
	Cross-sectional	Examines variables and relationships at one time point
	Retrospective	Retraces participants with an outcome backwards to a possible exposure
	Case-control	Cases matched to controls
	Cohort	Follows participants from exposure to outcome
	Longitudinal	Repeated measurements of participants over time
Quasi-experimental	Time-series	Manipulation (intervention)
	Non-equivalent control group	Manipulation + control
Experimental	After-only experimental	No measure prior to intervention
	Randomized controlled trial	Control & manipulation + random assignment to groups
	Cluster-randomized controlled trial	Groups of participants (not individuals) are randomized

Source: Schneider et al., (2016) *Nursing and Midwifery Research: methods and appraisal for evidence-based practice* 5th edn. Australia: Elsevier. Reproduced with permission.

MIXED METHODS APPROACHES

A third approach, mixed methods, has been defined as 'research in which the investigator collects and analyses data, integrates the findings, and draws inferences using both qualitative and quantitative approaches or methods in a single study or a program of inquiry' (Tashakkori and Creswell, 2007: 4). Mixed methods research is increasing in popularity (Creswell, 2014), despite challenges to the idea that mixed methods research is a coherent paradigm (Harrits, 2011); and that the development and progress of this paradigm is being hindered by the observation that qualitative and quantitative findings may not be fully integrated (Bryman, 2007). A further development in this methodology is methodological triangulation in mixed methods research (e.g. simultaneous, sequential transformative), each combination playing a part in altering the design.

A new framework for validating mixed methods research studies was developed by Dellinger and Leech (2007) and Leech et al. (2010), who argue that the term qualitative and quantitative research 'grossly oversimplifies what are rich and complex traditions, ideas, approaches, and techniques of research' (Dellinger and Leech, 2007, p 309). Researchers undertaking mixed methods research will encounter increased demands on their knowledge of philosophical and conceptual differences between qualitative and quantitative research approaches regarding study design, data collection and data analysis. What is clear is that researchers who choose to use some type of mixed methods design do so in the hope that they will produce data about their topic that are more comprehensive and integral.

Pfaff et al. (2014) used a mixed methods approach to explore new graduate nurse confidence in interprofessional collaboration. New graduate nurses from Ontario, Canada ($n = 514$) completed a cross-sectional descriptive survey that measured perceived confidence in interprofessional collaboration. Follow-up qualitative telephone interviews were conducted with 16 participants. The quantitative findings suggested that several factors had a positive relationship with nurse confidence; the qualitative phase supported these findings.

JUSTIFICATION OF THE RESEARCH APPROACH AND METHODS

The characteristic that makes an investigation a research inquiry, rather than simply an investigation of a problem in one setting, is the ability of the researcher to use the study findings to add new understanding of the problem beyond that one setting. The publishers of research journals will instruct researcher authors to address this aspect by having them state the following:

- What is already known about this topic?
- What does this study add to this topic?

Research review committee members will want to know how a study will add new understanding, and this is often referred to as the 'so what?' question. In other words the following questions may be asked:

So what new or additional information and understanding is your study contributing to what we already know? If it is not adding anything new, then why should your study be conducted?

How does a researcher ensure that she or he is adding to what is already known? This is achieved by describing a gap in our knowledge about the problem with reference to either the existing theory, or, if not a theory, at least a conceptual framework. This was covered in Step Two (Background and Justification for the Study). One of the next tasks of Step Three (Research Approach and Design) is to use this gap in our theoretical or conceptual understanding as the basis and rationale for the choice of research design and the subsequent methods.

Students undertaking higher degrees in the health sciences are often confused and apprehensive about the necessity or desirability of using a theoretical or conceptual framework in their research study. There is a clear distinction between a *theoretical* framework and a *conceptual* framework. A theoretical framework is one that uses or represents a known theory, for instance, Piaget's Theory of Child Development. A theoretical framework clearly implies using an existing theory and one that can provide a strong scientific base for a study, for instance, the connection of the researcher to existing knowledge. Ip, Tang and Goggins (2009) used Bandura's self-efficacy theory as the basis for an efficacy-enhancing educational intervention programme to improve women's ability to cope with childbirth. A detailed discussion on theoretical frameworks can be found on the University of Southern California Libraries Research Guides website (https://libraries.usc.edu).

A conceptual framework refers to 'the conceptual status of the things being studied, and their relationship to each other' (Punch, 2006: 49). This type of framework is one determined by the researcher who decides how the research question will be investigated, that is, the type and number of concepts to be explored, for instance, exploring women's perceptions of anxiety and fear. It specifies the way the study will be conducted. Bourke et al. (2012) developed a conceptual framework of six concepts of rural and remote health in Australia. Whether it is appropriate or advisable to use either a theoretical or conceptual framework in your study is something that needs to be discussed with your supervisor. For example, in many qualitative research approaches, stating a conceptual or theoretical framework is not necessary because the philosophy that underpins the particular research approach is implicit. In grounded theory, the theoretical framework 'evolves during the research itself' (Strauss and Corbin, 1990, p 49).

COMMENT ON USE OF A CONCEPTUAL FRAMEWORK

Natasha and Liang are both using conceptual frameworks. To illustrate this let us look back at the concept maps and literature reviews of Natasha (Figure 2.1) and Liang (Figure 2.2) in Step 2 and then answer the following five questions:

- What does the researcher want to investigate?
- What conceptual framework has the researcher described?
- How can the conceptual framework guide the research approach and methods?
- What do we know?
- What don't we know – what is the gap and hence appropriate study design?

NATASHA'S STUDY

What does she want to investigate?

- Pregnant women's anxiety and fear in the first trimester.
- How pregnant women cope with their feelings.

She wants to understand the women's interpretation and meaning of what anxiety and fear mean to them and so she has not provided a definition of anxiety or fear.

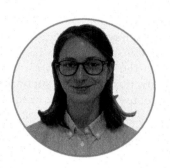

What conceptual framework has she described?

Natasha has drawn a framework of six core concepts surrounding the woman's anxiety and fear. Two of these concepts seem to be the descriptions of the actual experience, these being '"living" the pregnancy' and 'coping strategies'. Two concepts seem to be the woman's internal responses to the experience, these being 'attitude to pregnancy' and 'locus of control'. Two other concepts were considered important: (a) the support available to the woman, and (b) whether the pregnancy was planned or unplanned.

Natasha has also argued that pregnancy is a 'normal and natural' life event and the notion of wellbeing underlies and reinforced this view.

HOW CAN THE CONCEPTUAL FRAMEWORK GUIDE NATASHA'S RESEARCH APPROACH AND METHODS?

These six concepts have the potential to guide Natasha in making a decision about the participant profile. In the first instance, Natasha would not plan her recruitment on the basis of those women (and their partners) who planned or did not plan their pregnancy. This kind of information will emerge from the interview itself. Natasha feels that a question about not planning a pregnancy could have a negative connotation and involve questions of religious belief and partner relationship for the woman, who might then ask herself, 'should I have planned my pregnancy?'

When Natasha develops interview questions, the six concepts that she has identified (see Figure 2.1) could guide what she seeks to ask them. Given that there have also been previous studies on the topic, albeit not in the first trimester, it would be appropriate to use one or more available questionnaire instruments from these previous studies thereby enabling comparison with the findings of these studies.

Having identified wellbeing as a relevant concept, Natasha can focus on this when interviewing women about their coping strategies. That is, it is not just about coping, but coping to achieve a sense of wellbeing and that does not necessarily mean an absence of anxiety and fear.

From this framework of concepts, the choice of a mixed methods study can be argued as appropriate to answer the research question.

WHAT DO WE KNOW?

Much research literature presents pregnancy as a period of upheaval and a potential crisis state where stress and anxiety can lead to adverse birth outcomes. This leads to the justification for a study that identifies these stresses, anxieties and coping strategies so that supportive interventions can be provided. Previous studies have focused on women in the second and third trimesters.

What don't we know – what is the gap and hence appropriate study design?

From the review of the research literature, Natasha has logically concluded that the earlier a woman's anxieties and fears can be assuaged, the greater the likelihood of a better birth experience and outcome. Hence a study that is focused on low-risk women, pregnant for the first time (primigravidae), in the first trimester is argued as warranted and is the gap to be filled.

The women in Natasha's study are primigravidae. Natasha wanted to avoid the possible effects of past pregnancy experiences by evoking negative or positive emotions and so influencing the experience of the present pregnancy. The qualitative nature of the proposed study would, however, enable these questions to be explored in an interview, and along with the suggested use of a questionnaire instrument from previous studies, the use of a mixed methods study appears to have been justified and informed by Natasha's conceptual framework.

LIANG'S STUDY

What does he want to investigate?

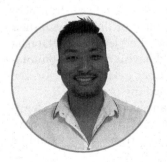

Liang wants to test an intervention of collaborative care in General Practice for people with co-morbid depression and heart disease and/or diabetes that:

- leads to positive client outcome, and
- is feasible within the role and skill capacity of nurses in a General Practice team as well as within current Australian health care system funding.

What conceptual framework has he described?

Liang has drawn a concept map as a series of concentric circles, with the client at the centre, moving out to the General Practice team (shown as the GP and the nurse), then to the system of care that is made up of four elements. Around these concentric circles are resources (funding and training) and the conceptual understandings of co-morbidity and collaborative practice, implying that these are relevant factors in the wider environment outside of the General Practice.

How can the conceptual framework guide Liang's research approach and methods?

The concentric nature of circles within the General Practice care system, with linked factors on the periphery, suggests research methods that will collect data about that system of care and how the factors interrelate to produce the client outcomes. At this point in the proposal development, Liang has not yet described the outcomes that he wants to measure.

The testing of an intervention against client outcomes suggests that an experimental design would be appropriate, as this can measure if those who receive the intervention score better than those who do not. The question of feasibility within role and skill capacity could suggest a qualitative approach, related to team members' experience, whereas feasibility related to funding suggested an economic analysis.

What do we know?

The adverse impact of co-morbid chronic disease is identified, with General Practice being the usual setting where chronic disease management takes place. Research is cited showing that multifaceted interventions are beneficial, but that GPs need a collaborative team-based system of care in order to manage the complex care needs of clients with co-morbidities.

The introduction of new funding for chronic disease management is stated as providing the opportunity to test the feasibility of a collaborative team-based system of care within the new level of funding.

What don't we know – what is the gap and hence appropriate study design?

An implied gap is stated in the need to know if changes can be made in the system of chronic disease care in General Practice using the new level of funding. There is a connection to 'collaborative practice' being a concept where those in the General Practice team might work together, using evidence-based guidelines reported in the international literature. Hence the study appears to be one that takes proven strategies for team-based chronic disease management to see if these can be feasibly applied in the Australian GP team and funding context. The particular gap that is identified is the focus on co-morbid chronic diseases, whereas most previous studies have focused on single disease management.

A mixed methods study would be appropriate to guide data collection and analysis across the two research questions. First, an experimental design would be appropriate to test the effectiveness of the team-based intervention, possibly drawing on instruments used in previous studies. This could include some economic analysis of the costs balanced against the funding received to determine funding feasibility. Second, a qualitative component (perhaps using interviews) would be appropriate to describe the experience of those involved in the collaborative team-based care to determine skill and capacity feasibility. Given that the client comprises the central circle in the conceptual framework, it would also be appropriate to understand their experience of the intervention.

DEFINING AND OPERATIONALIZING CONCEPTS FOR DATA COLLECTION

Regardless of the study it is important, to varying extents, to define and operationalize the concepts about which data are to be collected and analysed. This defining and operationalizing follows on from the previous task in the research design step where the study concepts were identified through a framework. However, simply naming concepts like anxiety and fear, or care team roles, or levels of depression, does not specify what data are to be collected. In the case of Natasha's study, it appears that she wants to leave the defining and operationalizing of her main concepts reasonably open so that the women participants are able to freely respond in an interview about what anxiety and fear they have experienced and what these terms mean to them. The following excerpts from Natasha's and Liang's proposals explain their rationale for the definitions they used to operationalize their concepts.

COMMENT ON EXCERPT FROM NATASHA'S AND LIANG'S PROPOSALS EXPLAINING THEIR OPERATIONALIZATION OF STUDY CONCEPTS

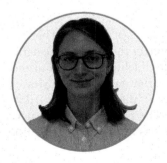

The aim of Natasha's study is to identify situations and events which cause anxiety and fear in the first trimester of pregnancy; the objective is to obtain uniquely personal, rich data through in-depth interviews using a qualitative approach. She has specified the grounded theory method of qualitative data collection and data analysis, as well as administration of the 'Ways of Coping Questionnaire (WCQ)', a self-report questionnaire (Folkman and Lazarus, 1988).

The purpose of a grounded theory study is to understand the feelings, behaviour and actions of individuals and to explain the merging patterns of behaviour of a higher level of abstraction that is, a theory (Chenitz and Swanson, 1986). This type of research adopts an '*emic*' approach or insider's point of view (Spradley, 1979), and affords an inside perspective of the women's perceptions of their experiences of anxiety and fear, and the meanings they attach to those experiences, as they themselves *experience* them.

Natasha does not want to prescribe a definition of anxiety and fear. In the case of coping strategies, the questionnaire (Ways of Coping Questionnaire – WCQ) provides, at least partly, a definition of those things measured in the instrument. If Natasha were also to ask open-ended questions about coping in the interview, then this concept would not only be limited to interpretations covered in the questionnaire.

In the interview, the concept of planned and unplanned pregnancy would be explained simply as 'did you make a decision about the timing of your pregnancy?' or 'was your pregnancy unplanned?' This would enable any differences in women's experience to be about that experience, not because of a different understanding of what 'planned and unplanned' meant.

For other studies, such as Liang's, where measurement is a key feature of the research design, measures of client outcome, such as levels of depression, diabetes and heart disease need to be specified. In the 'Nuts and Bolts' section below, the following study concepts are defined and operationalized in detail by virtue of what is being used for the measures, such as the PHQ-9 instrument as an indicator of depression and HbA1c scores as an indicator of diabetes control. Because there is a large list, it has been helpful to show these in a table (see Table 3.4 on p. 69). Broadly, Liang has grouped the operational concepts under the following categories:

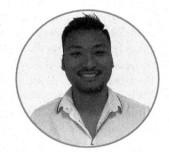

- Training programme evaluation.
- Feasibility of the model – skills and capacity.
- Client clinical outcomes.
- Feasibility of the model – funding.

THE 'NUTS AND BOLTS' – SAMPLING STRATEGIES/DATA COLLECTION/DATA ANALYSIS/ LIMITATIONS/DEMONSTRATING RIGOUR

We have called the methods section of a proposal the 'nuts and bolts' because this is the section where you describe what it is that you will actually do to achieve your data collection and analysis goals. Because most proposal templates provide a word or page limit for each section, the challenge is to provide sufficient detail about the methods within these limits. This is important in order for the committee members reviewing the proposal to understand what you want to do, and to judge if the methods appear to be rigorous. The committee members also need to see how the methods fit together and that the methods are logical. For this reason the use of tables and study diagrams can be helpful in conveying detailed and complex concepts in a minimum of page space.

Given that there are many research designs, there will equally be many ways to develop the methods for a study. A committee will want to be convinced that there is a logical fit between all of the steps in the proposal, these being: the problem being investigated and the associated theoretical or conceptual framework; the research question; the overall design, and the detailed methods. They will also want to know that you recognize the limitations of what you are proposing and that these limitations do not invalidate the worth of conducting the study. Finally, they will want to be assured that you and your team have the skills and resources to conduct the study. All these aspects of research design are dependent upon feasibility, which we will discuss in Step 5.

As a way of examining the logical fit of the methods section of a proposal, we have provided these sections of Natasha's and Liang's proposals. The activity in Read-Reflect-Respond 3.3 is for you to select at least one of these proposals (both if you feel so inclined), and consider how well Natasha or Liang has described their methods. You will also want to look at what they described in their previous Step Two (Background and Justification of the Study).

However, before you complete this activity there is one more section of Step Three to cover, which is about demonstrating the rigour of the design.

READ–REFLECT–RESPOND 3.3

CRITIQUE OF NATASHA'S AND LIANG'S METHODS

The methods section of both Natasha's and Liang's proposals are provided on the following pages. Select one (or both if you like), and using the material provided earlier by Natasha and Liang in this and the previous steps, review their methods section to determine if it is sufficient for a review committee to understand how the aspects of the study fit together into a coherent and logical research design that will answer the research question. There are many critical review guidelines for qualitative and quantitative studies; we have included two, one for qualitative studies and the other for quantitative studies, as Appendix A and Appendix B at the end of this book.

CHECKLIST FOR RESEARCH DESIGN

1.　Is there a theoretical or conceptual framework and, if so, how does this inform the study design and methods?
2.　Is the research design and reason for the approach clearly stated?
3.　Does the study design include aims and objectives (and hypotheses if appropriate) and are these suitable to address the research problem?
4.　Is the research question and/or objectives broken down into operational concepts for which data can be collected?

5. Do the study participants and the sampling strategy seem appropriate?
6. Do the data collection and data analysis techniques look to be rigorous according to the conventions of the study design?

DEMONSTRATING RIGOUR

A review committee will want to be assured that your study methods are of an acceptable standard so that they can be confident that the findings and inferences are research based. This is called the study rigour. Each research approach, and even each design within each approach, has accepted rigour conventions. One way to convince a review committee that your study is rigorous is to use the relevant convention terms and to demonstrate how these conventions are being applied in your study. There are too many designs and related conventions for us to cover in this Guide, but it will be helpful to describe these broadly across the quantitative and qualitative approaches. We will not specifically deal with mixed methods rigour here; however, the need to demonstrate rigour of a mixed methods study can be achieved with reference to the conventions that are described in related research texts and methodological journal articles (for instance, O'Cathain, 2009).

Quantitative rigour

Quantitative rigour requires the fulfilment of two conventions. The first is that the study findings can be accepted as being valid because the sample is representative of the population of interest and that the instruments have measured what they are supposed to measure (Last, 2001). This is called validity and, while there are many types of validity, the two main validation categories are internal and external validity. Internal validity is the confidence that the study methods are sound and that the researcher can infer that the association found between a predictor variable and an outcome variable is a valid inference and not likely to be because of some other factor – another untested variable, such as poor allocation of participants to the study groups, or because of a measurement problem. External validity is the confidence that the study sample is representative of a population that enables the researcher to infer that the study findings can be generalized to that population.

The second quantitative rigour convention is about reliability, which is the degree to which study methods are stable. Reliability means that if the study were repeated it would lead to the same (or very similar) findings. For example, when measuring weight or height, the same technique should be used for each participant. Hence the study may specify that these should be measured with the person unclothed so that different clothes and footwear do not contribute to different scores between participants, or between repeated measures with the same participants over time.

The threat to the validity and reliability of a quantitative study occurs when there is some bias in the methods. This occurs when the study methods cause a deviation in the findings that are systematically different from what is true (Last, 2001:14). While we do not know what is true – otherwise we would not be conducting the study – we do know if there is likely to be some bias in the methods. Where there is bias, we cannot confidently make inferences and conclusions about the findings.

Because there are many types of validity, reliability and bias, the researcher needs to consult research texts (see, for instance, Schneider at al., 2016, Chapters 10–13) and methodological journal articles so as to be aware of the relevant rigour issues pertinent to their study, and what strategies can be used to minimize these. In the proposal you should describe these issues and what steps are to be taken to ensure rigour and to minimize bias. However, because no one study is perfect you should also describe the limitations of the method. This will convey to the review committee that you are proposing the most rigorous study within your resources and capability, that you are aware of the limitations of the methods, and that your findings and inferences will be made with some caution in acknowledging these limitations.

Qualitative rigour

Qualitative rigour conventions are also numerous and these depend on the particular study design. Hence the qualitative researcher should consult relevant research texts (for instance, Schneider at al., 2016, Chapters 7–8) and methodological journal articles (e.g., Mays and Pope, 2000), and demonstrate in their proposal how the study rigour is to be assured.

Because qualitative studies do not seek to objectively measure the association between variables, but rather seek to explore subjectivities, the quantitative rigour concepts of validity, reliability and bias are not appropriate. We have described in Table 3.3 three qualitative rigour conventions that cover a spread of rigour issues relevant to many qualitative studies.

Table 3.3   Three common qualitative rigour conventions

Credibility	This is the degree to which the findings of a study and the claims made can be held as credible. Strategies that ensure 'information richness' and 'thick description' will mean that the findings have substance and that claims are not made on flimsy or shallow data. This is somewhat similar to the concept of validity.
Trustworthiness	This is the degree to which the methods of a study can be considered to have generated data that are consistent with the purpose of the study. For example if a study sought to determine participants' 'lived experiences' (phenomenology), then the sampling methods should purposively recruit participants who have had the experience of interest. Also, the methods of data collection and analysis should enable the participants' voices to be paramount.
Transferability	This is the manner in which the findings from a study can be considered to have relevance to settings and people beyond the immediate study. While not seeking to generalize, a qualitative researcher still needs to show how their findings and claims add to our understanding of the problem and how this may be useful to others. For example, when a researcher describes the context and conditions of their study this description can be used to also understand the problem in other settings under similar conditions and with similar people.

Important note

While we have indicated the need to demonstrate rigour, we have not actually described the numerous strategies that can be used to demonstrate this. There are simply too many techniques, and these are well described in research methods text books, but as an illustration of what we mean by demonstrating rigour we provide the following example. If a researcher wanted to claim that the findings of a study sample applied to a population (to generalize), then the sampling technique would need to show appropriate randomization techniques for participant selection so that the study can be considered as externally valid.

NATASHA'S METHODS SECTION

SAMPLE RECRUITMENT

The sample of primigravidae (pregnant for the first time) women and in their first trimester will be selected on the basis of theoretical sampling, that is, sample size will be determined by the data, and no additional participants will be sought once saturation has occurred and no new data will emerge. The concept of 'proven theoretical relevance' is important in grounded theory, meaning that concepts emerge as significant through their repeated presence or notable absence in the data (Strauss and Corbin, 1990: 176). The sample will be recruited from the antenatal clinic of hospital X. Women in the first trimester of their 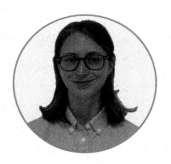 first pregnancy attending the clinic will be invited to participate in the study. Women who indicate their interest will be given a plain language information statement and consent form approved by the Faculty of Humanities and Social Sciences at University X and Hospital X. Issues of privacy and confidentiality will be clarified, and permission to tape record interviews will be sought. Natasha's contact phone number will be on the form. Any questions will be answered and an interview arranged in the women's respective homes.

DATA COLLECTION

In order to capture the essence of the women's experiences, a phenomenological or *lived experience* approach to data collection will also be used. An informal, open-ended interview, lasting about one hour, will be conducted. It is acknowledged that the interview between researcher and participant is an artificial situation. In order to minimize the artificiality aspect, the following techniques will be used: the setting is a natural environment (in the woman's home), the topic is familiar, and plain language will be used.

The meaning and interpretation a woman gives to events in her pregnancy are uniquely hers and become a source of discovery, of new information, rather than verifying other women's experiences. In this sense, a qualitative approach is contextual research, that is, the social world of the woman (both setting and phenomenon) has the best chance of being captured. A broad opening question could be 'Describe how you feel when you are anxious or frightened'. This would lead into their experiences of anxiety and fear in the first trimester.

DATA ANALYSIS

The first analytic step is open coding and the reduction of data into concepts concurrent with the constant comparative method. Coded data will then be grouped to form categories. Data will be coded as follows: open coding with memo writing assisting in defining patterns and relationships between codes; axial coding to identify relationships; and selective coding to generate core categories. During data analysis memos will be written and open and theoretical coding employed.

LIANG'S METHODS SECTION

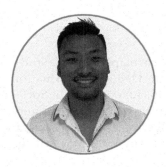

This project will complete a programme of work so that a model of collaborative care can be developed for clients with co-morbid depression and heart disease and/or diabetes. The study design is a cluster-randomized implementation trial. The trial does not aim to test the efficacy or effectiveness of the model of collaborative care, but rather to test that the model can be implemented under current Australian conditions in General Practice.

OBJECTIVES

1. To develop and test a training programme for nurses in General Practice in the screening, assessment and management of depression in clients with heart disease and/or diabetes.
2. To test the outcomes and feasibility of nurses to screen, assess, collect data, counsel, refer, review and monitor clients with co-morbid depression and heart disease and/or diabetes that can be funded using the new Medicare Benefits Schedule (MBS) Item Numbers.

INTERVENTION

1. Each General Practice database will be used to identify clients with diagnosed diabetes or heart disease. These clients will be invited to be screened for depression using the PHQ-9. Clients scoring above 5 (indicating mild or more severe depression) will be invited to participate in the study.
2. The evidence-based guidelines for management of diabetes, heart disease and depression are already available and Practices will be supported to turn these into useful computerized protocols and templates. These will be the basis for three-monthly client recall and checks carried out by the case manager (nurse).
3. The results of the chronic disease and depression risk assessments will be entered into an electronic database so that clinical audit and feedback of information to the practitioners can occur.
4. Case managers (nurses) working with the General Practices will be trained to manage mild depression using motivational interviewing, problem solving, promotion of physical activity and telephone counselling support. The case management team, led by the GP, will take overall responsibility for care planning, intervention and follow-up of clients with subclinical depression.
5. Clients with moderate to severe depression will be referred to existing mental health services in the region. Each practice will be assisted to develop close links with relevant services.
6. In all cases the case management team ensures that the client does not get lost in the system or drop out of treatment. The Practice database will provide the mechanism for routine follow-up of these clients.

SAMPLE

General practitioners and practice nurses working in 18 General Practices will be recruited from urban and rural regions from two Australian states. The criteria for selecting practices are: (1) the existing use of an electronic client database with the ability to identify those with diabetes or heart disease, (2) the availability of a nurse working in the General Practice, and (3) agreement to use the collaborative model of care.

From the 18 General Practices, nine will be randomly allocated to receive the intervention initially, and then the remaining nine General Practices will serve as a wait list control (they will receive the intervention after the controlled trial is completed).

It is estimated that a sample of 450 clients will be required from nine General Practices in the intervention group and nine in the control group. The sample size calculation is based on detecting a 50% reduction in depression score at the 0.05 significance level with 80% power under a two-tailed test and allowing for a 50% drop out. Because randomization is by Practice, an intra-cluster correlation of 0.04

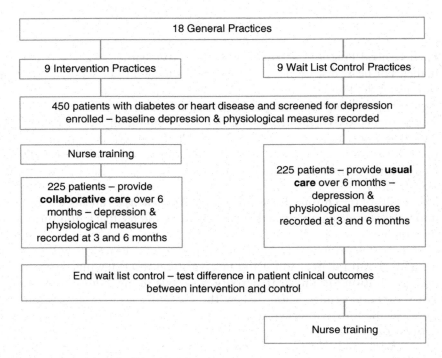

Figure 3.1   Liang's study flowchart

has also been applied. A recruitment target of 50 clients per General Practice has been set so that a nurse can carry out the intervention with four to five clients each week over the three-month cycle of care.

The study flowchart is shown in Figure 3.1 above.

DATA COLLECTION

The instruments to be used are the following:

- Training programme evaluation – pre-, post- and 3-month follow-up question-naire (to be adapted from National Heart Foundation of Australia Depression Workshops).
- The Patient Health Questionnaire 9 (PHQ-9) which is a validated instrument to detect depression in the general population.
- Audit tool for baseline and follow-up data on feasibility and client clinical outcomes.
- Structured interview schedule for research assistant interview with GPs, practice nurses and clients at end of project.

How these will be used is described in Table 3.4 below.

Table 3.4   Liang's study – data items

OUTCOME DATA ITEM	SOURCE
Training program evaluation	
Pre- and post-test of knowledge and confidence.	Questionnaire administered prior to and at end of training programme.
Confidence and capacity to use training materials.	Questionnaire administered via telephone three months after training programme.
Feasibility of the model – skills and capacity	
Baseline data on current practice – proportion of clients who have previously had physiological and depression risk factors recorded (e.g. lipids, BP, smoking status, depression score, etc.).	Document what GPs and PNs currently do – questionnaire during training programme. Baseline clinical data derived from General Practice database.
Number/proportion of recalled clients for whom collaborative management plan has been completed (including management of depression where relevant).	Derived from management plan.
Number/proportion of clients who are monitored, recalled and reassessed using PHQ-9.	
Number/proportion of clients referred to community resources.	
Acceptability of enhanced role of practice nurses in depression screening and assessment, case management, review, monitoring and referral of clients.	Structured interview at end of project.
Client clinical outcomes	
Client satisfaction with collaborative chronic disease management model including enhanced role of practice nurse.	Structured interview at end of project.
HbA1c, lipids, platelet inhibitor use, blood pressure, smoking status, physical activity, weight management results.	Derived from client & practice records.
Changes in PHQ-9 scores – number/proportion of clients identified with mild/moderate/severe depression.	
Number/proportion of clients for whom mental health plan was included in the collaborative management plan.	
Number/proportion of clients referred, or recommended, by nurse to community resources.	
Feasibility of the model – funding	
Number of relevant Medicare Benefit Schedule Items billed via this process.	Derived from client & practice records.
Estimated GP, nurse and administration time per client visit in each participating practice – profitability compared to usual care.	Structured interview at end of project.
Barriers, enablers and ways to improve system.	Structured interview at end of project.

DATA ANALYSIS

In order to compare the effectiveness of the model to the usual-care control, ANCOVAs will be used to adjust for baseline values and test the significance of changes in continuous variables between the two groups after six months. A multilevel mixed-effects logistic regression will be used to test the significance of changes in the binary (categorical) variables between the two groups after six months. Within each group, changes between the two time points (baseline and six-month visits) will be tested using paired t-tests for the continuous variables and matched-case-control McNemar χ^2 tests for the binary variables.

The longer-term effects of the intervention will be evaluated over the 12-month period using multilevel mixed-effects linear regression for the continuous variables and multilevel mixed-effects logistic regression for the binary variables. All three-monthly data available in the intervention group over the 12 months will be used. Note that the study design will not collect 'usual care' data from the control clinics beyond six months, after which they cease to be a control.

Acceptability of the model of collaborative care to the intervention group nurses, GPs and clients will be assessed qualitatively through interviews to be held at the completion of the study. All intervention group nurses and GPs will be invited to be interviewed, while 27 volunteer intervention group clients will be sought for interview (3 clients per clinic). It is assumed that by spreading client recruitment across the clinics and with a sample size of 27 clients, both maximum variation as well as data saturation will be achieved. Interviews will be digitally recorded, transcribed verbatim and thematically analysed to examine the following three broad themes:

- acceptability and feasibility of the enhanced nurse role;
- client satisfaction with the model of collaborative care;
- barriers and enablers to implementing the model and possible model improvements.

LIMITATIONS

For inclusion, the study will recruit only General Practices that use a clinical software database and have a nurse on staff. Hence Practices that chose to take part in the study may not be representative of wider General Practices.

Usual care in the control General Practices may be changed by clients completing the PHQ-9 and reading the project description. GPs in these control Practices will be made aware of individual PHQ-9 results and will likely take action where warranted. Hence GP awareness of these biophysical and lifestyle risks may be expected to change clinical management also in the control General Practices. This may lead to a smaller effect size difference and so an under estimation of the impact of the intervention.

CONCLUSION

The research design step in writing a research proposal is a big step. This is because it involves a description of the actual research activities along with the decision-making rationale about these activities. In this step we have identified the researchable question as the core from which design decisions are made. We have shown how it is beneficial to use a theoretical or conceptual framework as the basis from which to design a study and we have described when it is important to operationalize the study concepts to inform data collection and analysis.

In order to convince a review committee that a study is sound and worthwhile there needs to be a logical fit between all of the components of the research design. This includes declaring the limitations of the study and describing what techniques will be used to ensure rigour.

To conclude, before moving onto Step Four you can now move to the final activity in Step Three which is to write your own research design.

 ## ACTIVITY 3.1 RESEARCH DESIGN – STEP THREE

In Activity 2.2. you were asked to write the working title, background and justification for your proposal.

1. Restate the working title of your proposal and add the research question from Read-Reflect-Respond 3.1.
2. Using the checklist from Read-Reflect-Respond 3.3, write out your own research design.
3. Keep in mind the various qualitative and quantitative research approaches; indicate clearly which design you have chosen and give reasons for your choice.
4. If any one of the points in the checklist are omitted from your design, for example, 'theoretical or conceptual framework', indicate why you have not used one.

REVISION

Below you will find five statements related to the content of this chapter. Indicate whether you think each statement to be true or false. The answers are given on p. 74.

1. The first step in developing a research design is to ensure that you have a researchable question.

   T/F

2. While there are differences in the research approaches and purpose these should not influence the logic and rationale for the data collection and analysis.

   T/F

3. Using a theoretical or conceptual framework enables the findings of a study to have relevance beyond the immediate study setting and sample.

   T/F

4. The same rigour conventions apply to both qualitative and quantitative methods.

   T/F

5. Data collection in quantitative research should not be influenced by the researcher.

   T/F

REFERENCES

Biddix, J.P. (2009) Research Rundowns. (https://researchrundowns.com). [Last accessed 5 September 2017]

Bourke, L., Humphreys, J.S., Wakerman, J. and Taylor, J. (2012) Understanding rural and remote health: a framework for analysis. *Health & Place*, 18(3): 496–503.

Bryman, A. (2007) Barriers to integrating quantitative and qualitative research. *Journal of Mixed Methods Research*, 1(1): 8–22.

Chenitz, W.C. and Swanson, J.M. (1986) *From Practice to Grounded Theory*. USA: Addison-Wesley Publishing Company.

Creswell, J.W. (2014) *Research Design: Qualitative, quantitative, and mixed-methods approaches* 4th edn. International Student edition. Thousand Oaks, CA: Sage Publications.

Dellinger, A.B. and Leech, N.L. (2007) Toward a unified validation framework in mixed methods research. *Journal of Mixed Methods Research*, 1(4): 309–332.

Duke University (undated) ICS capstone seminar: formulating a research question. (http://guides.library.duke.edu/c.php?g=289688&p=1930772). [last accessed 5 September 2017]

Folkman, S. and Lazarus, R.S. (1988) *Ways of Coping Questionnaire*. Palo Alto, CA: Consulting Psychologists Press.

Gillespie, B.M. and Chaboyer, W. (2016) 'Assessing measuring instruments', in Z.Schneider, D. Whitehead, G Lobiondo-Wood and J. Haber (eds) *Nursing and Midwifery Research: methods and appraisal for evidence-based practice* 5th edn. Australia: Elsevier, pp. 198–209.

Glaser, B. and Strauss, A. (1967) *The Discovery of Grounded Theory: strategies for qualitative research*. Chicago: Aldine.

Goodson, L. and Vassar, M. (2011) An overview of ethnography in healthcare and medical education research. *Journal of Educational Evaluation for Health Professions*, 8: 4.

Harrits, G.S. (2011) More than method? A discussion of paradigm differences within mixed methods research. *Journal of Mixed Methods Research*, 5(2): 150–166.

Ip, W-Y., Tang, C.S. and Goggins, W.B. (2009) An educational intervention to improve women's ability to cope with childbirth. *Journal of Clinical Nursing*, 18(15): 2125–2135.

Laffin, N., Smyth, W., Heyer, E., Fasugba, O., Abernethy, G. and Gardner, A. (2015) Effectiveness and acceptability of a moisturizing cream and a barrier cream during radiation therapy for breast cancer in the tropics. A randomized controlled trial. *Cancer Nursing*, 38(3): 205–214.

Last, J. (ed.) (2001) *A Dictionary of Epidemiology* 4th edn. Oxford University Press.

Leech, N.L., Dellinger, A.B., Brannagan, K.B. and Tanaka, H. (2010) Evaluating mixed research studies: a mixed methods approach. *Journal of Mixed Methods Research*, 4(1):17–31.

Mays, N. and Pope, C. (2000) Assessing quality in qualitative research. *BMJ*, 320: 50–52.

Mjaaland, T.A., Finset, A., Jensen, B.F. and Gulbrandsen, P. (2011) Patients' negative emotional cues and concerns in hospital consultations: a video-based observational study. *Patient Education & Counseling*, 85(3): 356–362.

O'Cathain, A. (2009) Mixed methods research in the health sciences. *Journal of Mixed Methods Research*, 3(1): 3–6.

Pfaff, K.A., Baxter, P.E., Jack, S.M. and Ploeg, J. (2014) Exploring new graduate nurse confidence in interprofessional collaboration: a mixed methods study. *International Journal of Nursing Studies*, 51(8): 1142–1152.

Pope, C. (2005) Conducting ethnography in medical settings. *Medical Education*, 39(12): 1180–1187.

Punch, K.F. (2006) *Developing Effective Research Proposals* 2nd edn. London: Sage Publications.

Queensland University of Technology (undated) IFN 001 Advanced information research skills (AIRS): How to formulate a good research question. (http://airs.library.qut.edu.au/resources/1/1). [last accessed 5 September 2017]

Sbaraini, A., Carter, S.M., Evans, R.W. and Blinkhorn, A. (2011) How to do a grounded theory study: a worked example of a study of dental practices. *BMC Medical Research Methodology*, 11: 128.

Schneider, Z., Whitehead, D., LoBiondo-Wood, G. and Haber, J. (eds) (2016) *Nursing and Midwifery Research: methods and appraisal for evidence-based practice* 5th edn. Chatswood, Australia: Elsevier.

Shields, L. and Smyth, W. (2016) 'Common qualitative approaches', in Z. Schneider., D. Whitehead, G. Lobiondo-Wood and J. Haber (eds) *Nursing and Midwifery Research: methods and appraisal for evidence-based practice* 5th edn. Australia: Elsevier, pp. 143–164.

Spradley, J.P. (1979) *The Ethnographic Interview*. Fort Worth, TX: Holt, Harcourt Brace, Jovanovich Publishers.

Strauss, A. and Corbin, J. (1990) *Basics of Qualitative Research: Grounded Theory Procedures and Techniques*. Newbury Park, CA: Sage Publications.

Tashakkori, A. and Creswell, J.J. (2007) Editorial: The new era of mixed methods. *Journal of Mixed Methods Research*, 1(1): 3–7.

Taylor, S.J. and Bogdan, R. (1984) *Introduction to Qualitative Research Methods* 2nd edn. New York, NY: Wiley.

University of Southern California. Organising Your Social Science Research Paper: Theoretical Framework. (http://libguides.usc.edu/writingguide/theoreticalframework). [accessed 5 September 2017]

Van Manen, M. (1990) *Researching Lived Experience: human science for an action sensitive pedagogy*. London, Ontario: Althouse.

Winger, A., Ekstedt, M., Wyller, V.B. and Helseth, S. (2013) 'Sometimes it feels as if the world goes on without me': adolescents' experiences of living with chronic fatigue syndrome. *Journal of Clinical Nursing*, 23(17–18): 2649–2657.

ANSWERS TO ACTIVITIES

 READ–REFLECT–RESPOND 3.1

RESEARCH QUESTIONS

NATASHA'S research question could also specify:

- If these are primigravidae or not
- If these women are from particular groups, such as ethnic or age groups
- The research approach, e.g. a qualitative study or a grounded theory study.

LIANG's research question could also specify:

- Type of health conditions
- Type of patients
- Country (important for funding issues)

REVISION

1. T
2. F
3. T
4. F
5. T

STEP FOUR

CAPTURING ATTENTION– ABSTRACT, TITLE AND SIGNIFICANCE

CONTENT

- How to write a detailed abstract that captures attention
- Identifying a descriptive, concise and interesting title
- How to show that the outcomes will be significant
- Structuring for clarity to capture attention
- The art of culling words

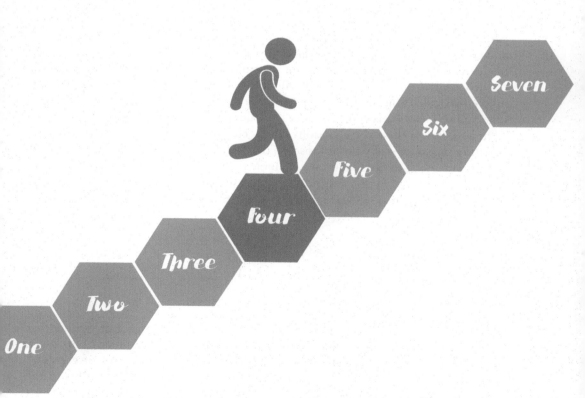

KEY TERMS/CONCEPTS

- Significance of outcomes
- Language level of layperson
- Active voice
- Consistent layout of concepts
- Judicious use of white space

INTRODUCTION

This chapter provides information about how to construct those sections of the proposal that will capture the attention of the committee. The three sections covered in this chapter can help you to sell your proposed research. These sections are the abstract (or synopsis), the title, and the study significance. These sections should be bold and hard hitting, but based in facts so that you are not seen to be overinflating the importance and likely value of your study. Nothing will turn review committee members off more than claims made about your research that cannot be seen in factual description in the proposal. It is not good enough to claim that your study is important – you need to show how it is important to the review committee.

The first sections of your proposal that the committee will read are the title and abstract and, as with any introduction, these should be carefully approached and prepared in order to make the desired impact, that is, to make them want to read your proposal. As a review committee will have many proposals to read through, you want to be sure that your proposal captures their attention because it is clear and compelling. Also included in this chapter is a discussion about the importance of clearly describing the significance of the study, as this is a major 'selling' point of the proposal. If the study outcomes will not be significant to anyone then the committee may ask, 'Why should we approve the study if no one will benefit from the time and resources needed to conduct the study?'

In addition to these three sections in this chapter, we also look at how you can structure the content of your proposal so that the reader can easily understand what you are intending to do. Finally, we examine the art of culling words. Both of these techniques ensure that you can provide the essential information within the word limit and that it is a clear description without clutter.

HOW TO WRITE A DETAILED ABSTRACT THAT CAPTURES ATTENTION

An abstract or synopsis of a proposal is a brief and succinct piece of writing that summarizes the entire proposal. The abstract identifies the importance of the topic, the research aims and objectives (or research question), the evidence of gaps and omissions in the literature, the research design, and the anticipated benefits of the study. Whether you include references to the previous studies in the abstract is a personal preference, but it is generally not necessary as these should be described in more detail in the body of the proposal.

The function of the abstract is to provide the reader with a concise yet comprehensive written statement about the research project. A well written, clear, plain language summary is particularly important because this will be the first part of the proposal that committee members will read. Therefore, care should be exercised in using English that is devoid of technical jargon and in a style that can reasonably be understood by people unfamiliar with your particular discipline and research area. For instance, many funding and ethical review committees will have some lay members (individuals who do not have specialized knowledge of a subject) and so you should pitch the language at a level that a lay person could understand. We will come back to this point in the section on structuring for clarity.

The proposal template will guide you as to the appropriate length and specific requirements of the abstract. The length may be anything from 100 words but is not likely to be more than a half a page. In the event that no word limit is specified, it would be wise to restrict the abstract to half a page.

Although the abstract appears as one of the first requirements on the proposal template (after the title), it is usually written last when all other components of the proposal have been completed. This is because the abstract needs to succinctly summarize all of these components.

TOP TIP

Write the abstract when you have energy.

Be careful of proposal writing burnout when writing the abstract. Because you leave the writing of the abstract till the end when you are likely to be feeling tired, and because it is essentially a summary of already written work, it is tempting to rush a half-baked abstract. This is poor proposal writing practice. Wait until you have some energy to write the abstract to ensure that it contains all the essential information. The abstract is a crucial part of the proposal as it creates the first impression, as Mohan-Ram (2000) has described:

> Because the abstract is the first glimpse a reader gets of an application's worth, such oversights [not including all essential information] can raise unnecessary questions, and may even create the impression that the research plan itself may be incomplete.

ELEMENTS OF A PROPOSAL ABSTRACT

An abstract should do the following:

1. Provide a concise, clearly written statement about the topic and its significance in the field (why it is important to conduct this study and what knowledge gap the study will fill).

2. Identify the type of existing research on the topic; the methodological similarities and differences to your own study, and the methodological gap the study will fill.
3. Describe the study in terms of aims and objectives, research approach and design, in order to show how the gaps and omissions will be addressed.
4. State what significant outcomes the study will achieve.

READ–REFLECT–RESPOND 4.1

Let us now look at the abstracts of both of our researchers, Natasha and Liang. Use the four point checklist to identify the elements in both Natasha's and Liang's proposal abstracts and make suggestions for any improvement you think appropriate. See our response to this activity on pp. 86–8 of the chapter.

NATASHA'S ABSTRACT

Pregnancy is a life-changing and role-changing event in a woman's life; it is a *rite of passage*. When a woman discovers that she is pregnant can it generate feelings of bewilderment, joy, amazement, confusion, anxiety, fear and ambivalence. Physical changes, over which the woman has little control, cause discomfort; she often becomes emotionally labile, and may experience vagueness and memory impairment. Of significance to the woman are anxiety and fear of the unknown.

Physical, emotional and cognitive symptoms of pregnancy continue to be widely discussed and debated in the literature (Byrne et al., 2014; Darwin et al., 2015; Davis-Floyd, 1992; Gross & Pattison, 1995; Hall et al., 2009; Harvey, 1992; LeBlanc, 1999; Lewellyn-Jones, 1998; Schneider, 2002; Usher, 1990); however, exploring anxiety and fear in the first trimester of pregnancy has not been addressed. This is a stark omission because of the potential negative impact on the course of the pregnancy. Women's experiences of anxiety and fear need to be investigated so that they can be assisted in developing coping strategies to mitigate against the pernicious effects of these potentially disabling emotions. The studies reviewed had different research approaches, samples, times at which questionnaires or interviews were administered, and data collection and analysis strategies.

First-time pregnant women in their first trimester and attending an antenatal clinic at Hospital X will be invited to participate. In-depth interviews (about one hour) will be conducted with each woman in her home. In addition, each woman will complete a 'Ways of Coping Questionnaire (WCQ)', a self-report questionnaire (Folkman and Lazarus, 1988). Grounded theory will guide data collection and analyses.

An analysis of the data will provide the opportunity to design an intervention programme, e.g., an app for communication between a woman, her partner, and clinic staff. Another option is weekly group sessions of Mindfulness Based Childbirth Education (MBCE), to help instil confidence and increased awareness of situations that produce anxiety and fear. In addition, group activity will provide the occasion for the women to explore concepts of self-efficacy, self-esteem, and locus of control.

NOTE: the citations used in Natasha's abstract are not listed in the references as these are not relevant to the learning in this chapter.

LIANG'S ABSTRACT

Depression, diabetes and heart disease represent three of the leading disease burdens in Australia with all three conditions being identified as National Health Priority Areas. Coronary heart disease

(CHD) and diabetes frequently co-exist, and the impact of depression on both conditions has been shown to result in significantly worse mortality and morbidity outcomes as well as increases in health care costs. These chronic conditions are managed in the main in General Practice, and it is in this setting that the majority of patients seek help.

The international literature has shown that chronic illness care benefits from comprehensive and multifaceted health service delivery, and that General Practices are central to the success of coordinated chronic disease management (CDM). GPs often have limited time to manage the complex care needs of their patients and they could benefit from additional resources to help in CDM. The new Medicare Benefits Schedule (MBS) Chronic Disease Management Items introduced in July 2005 offer a potential solution but this requires changes in practice organization.

This research aims to: (1) develop and test a training programme for general practitioners and practice nurses in the screening, assessment and management of depression in patients with heart disease and/or diabetes; and (2) to test the feasibility of practice nurses screening, assessing, collecting data, counselling, referring, reviewing and monitoring patients with co-morbid depression and heart disease and/or diabetes. The design is a cluster-randomized intervention trial that will recruit 18 General Practices in order to generate 450 patients, with physiological, psychological and lifestyle measures taken at 3, 6 and 12 months. The primary clinical outcome will be a change in depression scores.

This project will lead to a tested model for assessment and treatment of co-morbid depression and heart disease and/or diabetes that is based both on sound research findings and the way that Australian General Practice is developing. The study will set up systems within General Practices to demonstrate how the care of co-morbid depression and heart disease and/or diabetes can be funded successfully using the new Medicare Benefits Schedule (MBS) Item Numbers.

YOUR OWN ABSTRACT

Using your experience in assessing these example abstracts now write your own abstract in no more than 500 words.

- -

IDENTIFYING A DESCRIPTIVE, CONCISE AND INTERESTING TITLE

It is useful to begin with a working title of your study even if this is not the final title that you will decide on. In the first instance, the working title provides the broad label for what the research is about. When the final title is decided, this should be carefully crafted and interesting to make an impact on the reader. The title should be as short as possible (concise), but long enough to inform the reader about the topic and possibly the type of study (descriptive).

The wording of the title depends upon the nature of the research, which is the topic, the research design and the sample. It may be that your interest is in safety in the workplace, such as particular injuries sustained through falls. The title should indicate specifically what and where the workplace is and what constitutes 'falls' and what 'injuries'. Committee members reviewing the proposal must have this concise yet detailed information immediately. A working title is useful as your initial frame of reference, but this may change as you begin to review the literature. You should be sufficiently open-minded and flexible to modify your title as you read the research literature and as you design your study. If this process is carefully observed, a clear, straightforward title will emerge.

The working title of Natasha's research study started out as:

An investigation into pregnant women's experiences of ambivalence, anxiety and fears in the first trimester of pregnancy, and how they cope with their feelings.

Her final title was:

Women's experiences of anxiety and fear in the first trimester of pregnancy: a qualitative study.

The working title of Liang's research study started out as:

Chronic disease management of co-morbid depression and heart disease and/or diabetes

His final title written as a question was:

Is practice nurse-led collaborative care effective in the management of depression for patients with heart disease or diabetes?

FEATURES OF A CLEAR TITLE

The title of the research provides a description of what the project is about. Therefore the title should be descriptive, clear, specific and unambiguous, economically worded, and provide the following information:

- study problem
- research approach or design
- topic variables or concepts being investigated
- sample or participants (gender, age, ethnic group, etc.).

READ–REFLECT–RESPOND 4.2

PART A – ASSESSING A TITLE

Read the following examples of two poorly worded project titles, and using the checklist above consider what information would improve the title.

1. An examination of the relationship between smoking and alcohol consumption in a sample of five hundred 18 year old male and female school students.
2. The effects of music on people with dementia.

PART B – IMPROVING A TITLE

Using the above checklist for titles, identify and add the missing information in the following titles. (Our suggestions appear on p. 88; your suggestions may be different.)

1. An investigation into the dietary habits of Aboriginal and Torres Strait Islander peoples.
2. Multi-measure pain assessment in women living with cancer.
3. Culturally-based health care practices of Zulus.
4. The experiences of postnatal women's use of telemedicine.
5. An exploration of the experiences of Cultural Safety Educators overseas.

After you have improved these practice titles, see what you can do to improve the working title of your proposal.

HOW TO SHOW THAT THE OUTCOMES WILL BE SIGNIFICANT

Consideration of a research proposal will not only be made on the scientific merit of the study design (Step 3), but also on the significance of the outcomes to improve or benefit patient care, protocols, policies, etc. That is, the outcomes of your research need to be significant for someone or something. In order for this to be significant, nations and organizations often set priorities about topics that they want to improve through research. For example the Australian Government (2017), in consultation with industry, government and researchers, has identified nine research priorities on the most important challenges facing Australia. The current priorities are: food, soil and water, transport, cybersecurity, energy, resources, advanced manufacturing, environmental change and health. The Research Councils UK (undated) have a list of four priorities for the Medical Research Council, which are: infections, brain health and dementia, prevention, and regenerating damaged tissue. The National Institutes of Health (undated) in the USA, through its 27 institutes and centres, has also established research priorities.

National research priorities are invariably broad and, for more specific direction, university faculties, health services, government departments and funding agencies will also have their own research priorities. If your application is to one of these organizations, it would help if you can show how your research incorporates one of these priorities. In addition to information provided on websites, organizations often have a research grants officer, or similar staff member, who can provide advice to prospective applicants. It is always a good idea to speak with this person about your research idea and to do this before starting to write the proposal.

When assessing significance for project grants the National Health and Medical Research Council (NHMRC) of Australia defines significance and innovation, and these together contribute 25% of the assessment weighting. The NHMRC (undated) define significance of expected outcomes as one or more of the following:

- advancing knowledge in the field
- having an impact on health
- being of interest to other researchers and policy makers.

The NHMRC define innovation as one or more of the following:

- new, novel or creative
- cutting edge
- resulting in a paradigm shift
- affecting current practices or approaches
- describes new ideas, procedures, technologies, programmes or health policy settings
- yielding influential publications or invited international presentations.

Many proposal templates will have a section on significance. Even if they do not, the background section of a proposal should address the significance of the problem and the gap in knowledge. Then, in the most appropriate section in the proposal, you should describe how the research outcomes will help to address this problem.

READ–REFLECT–RESPOND 4.3

CRITIQUE THE SIGNIFICANCE SECTION OF LIANG'S PROPOSAL BEFORE WRITING YOUR OWN.

Below is the significance section of Liang's proposal. While reading this significance section, consider which of the NHMRC components of significance and innovation Liang has addressed in his proposal. We have marked up those sections that we consider deal with these.

This project will develop, test and implement a model for assessment and treatment that is based both on sound research findings and the way that Australian General Practice is developing the care of chronic illness. Programmes like *More Allied Health Services* and *Better Outcomes in Mental Health Care Initiative* provide opportunities for GPs to be better trained and to make referrals to these services. This project, which is aligned with the consultation draft of the National Chronic Disease Strategy, the National Service Improvement Framework for Diabetes and the National Service Improvement Framework for Heart, Stroke and Vascular Disease will also train the extended team, within and outside the General Practice to manage an integrated shared care model which can be sustained under the MBS CDM items introduced in July 2005. Our approach uses the world's best model for delivery of CDM including evidence-based guidelines and interprofessional teamwork in General Practice.

> Will be of interest to policy makers.

> Builds on existing evidence.

The programme uses the existing workforce but involves an enhanced role for the practice nurses and so is applicable for wider roll out in using these potentially under-utilized staff. The practice nurses will gain enhanced skills in the CDM set up and management that will be a useful model for patients with other chronic diseases.

> Significance of outcomes for nurses and patients. Innovation in possibly changing nurses' practice.

A full range of outcome measures will be reported and added to the electronic medical database. Consequently, Practices will know what happens to patients (process of care) and will be able to identify changes in classic risk factors, depression symptoms and affordability within the Australian health system.

> Significance for General Practices. Innovation in possibly changing practices in the clinic.

Having reviewed the significance section of Liang's proposal now write the significance section of your own proposal.

Congratulations! You have now completed Step Four of your proposal. As a first draft, however, the proposal is not likely to be clear and easy to read. The logic in the argument might be a little jumbled. Like any piece of writing it will need to be worked over a few times to get it polished so that it will capture and keep the attention of the committee members who will read it. The next two sections should help you with the polishing needed to capture and sustain the committee members' attention.

STRUCTURING FOR CLARITY TO CAPTURE ATTENTION

In addition to writing a compelling research design following on from an interesting research question that deals with an important problem, there are written language and layout techniques that you can use to help make your proposal clear and easy to read.

WRITTEN LANGUAGE

We have found that the following written language techniques can improve the 'readability' of a proposal.

- The use of an active voice in writing is one of the best ways to communicate what you intend to do. By active voice we mean that the subject (person) performs the action of the verb (e.g. the student *wrote* the proposal), as opposed to the passive voice where the subject (person) is acted *upon* or passive (e.g. the proposal *was written* by the student). Depending upon which form, active or passive, we use we can emphasize certain words. In the first example, the student is emphasized; in the second example, the proposal is emphasized. In general, the active voice is more direct and forceful than the passive voice.
- Use appropriate terminology because it is important to convey confidence to the reader that you have expertise in the topic of the research and also in research methods. However, do not overdo the use of highly technical language, as the reader could interpret this as you simply trying to impress, or trying to cover up a weak research design. Also if you use too much highly technical language then the reader may not understand you.
- Sell your idea and be a little bold, but also be realistic about what you claim your research will achieve. Being a little bold can convey a sense of confidence that you will achieve what you say you will; however, if you make claims that are too bold and unrealistic the reader will most likely pick this up and dismiss your application.

LAYOUT

In addition to what you write, how you lay the text out on the page is also important to improve 'readability'. Here are a few techniques that we use:

- Be consistent in how you order the concepts. For example, if you have three objectives, consider laying out the objectives in the sequence in which they will be addressed, then make sure that you lay text out that relates to these objectives in the same order that you have written them. Be consistent with this ordering throughout the proposal; this will help the reader to follow your text.
- Make judicious use of white space and avoid the temptation to cram a lot of words into the space provided on a template. This is less of a problem when maximum word counts are specified, but can be a trap when the limits are set as pages. When a researcher has a lot to describe, the temptation is to describe it all and in detail in order to convince the reader. Simply put, too much crammed text is too much. We remember a proposal from a computer scientist where there were no paragraph breaks at all, and this made the proposal very difficult to read. White space on a page provides a visual break between sections of text and this enables the reader's eye to differentiate these sections.
- Use visual aids, such as bullet points, tables and diagrams. While these visual aids can take up valuable space in the proposal, it would be a mistake not to consider using these as a good diagram can convey a lot of information to the reader about the research design and the relationship between the study components. Figure 3.1 is an example that shows the how the components of Liang's study have been represented in a diagram. One of the most commonly used visual aids in a research proposal is a Gantt Chart that shows the list of research activities and the sequence and duration of each activity.

THE ART OF CULLING WORDS

Focus your reader! Too many words are a distraction. Ask yourself these questions: 'Does this word add to the point I'm making?'; 'Can I say this more succinctly and keep the reader's attention and interest?' If you can convey the same message using only the most relevant words, then your words will have more power. Using fewer words is more efficient for the reader and so they are likely to understand more quickly what you want to say. For example, if you find a very large number of articles that relate to your topic, it may be necessary to do a 'cull' of the articles so that only those specifically related to your topic and design are read. The same applies to culling words from your writing; it amounts to choosing or selecting the best, most appropriate words to get your message across. If a research template has word limits then you may have to rework your text over a number of drafts so that you can convey what is needed within the word limits.

 ## READ–REFLECT–RESPOND 4.4

CULLING WORDS IN NATASHA'S ABSTRACT

Natasha's abstract (on p. 78) is 320 words, which is a reasonable length for an abstract. What if the proposal template, however, had a limit of 300 words or even 250 words? Can you cull

Natasha's abstract but still keep all the essential information? Once you have tried this, go to p. 89 to see how we have 'culled' some words in the abstract to within a 250 word limit.

CONCLUSION

This chapter has covered the steps required for your proposal to capture the attention of the review committee. While the research design (Step 3) is the 'engine room' of a research proposal, this will not be the first section that the committee will read. The title and abstract need to stimulate interest in the committee so they want to read more. It is important to argue that your anticipated research outcomes will have significant benefits to make the proposal worth approving. In the next step we consider whether your research is worth doing and your, and your team's, capacity to complete the research you are proposing.

REVISION

Below you will find five statements related to the content of this chapter. Indicate whether you think each statement to be true or false. The answers are given on p. 89.

1. You should never use technical language in a proposal because the review committee may not understand it.

   T/F

2. It is OK to make bold claims about the proposed research as long as these are grounded in some facts.

   T/F

3. Concepts should be laid out in the same order throughout the proposal.

   T/F

4. Reducing font size in a proposal is a good idea because you can then add much more detailed content.

   T/F

5. The abstract is usually written after the proposal has been completed.

   T/F

REFERENCES

Australian Government (2017) Science and research priorities. (www.science.gov.au/scienceGov/ScienceAndResearchPriorities/Pages/default.aspx). [last accessed 27 August 2017]

Mohan-Ram, V. (2000) Abstract killers: how not to kill a grant application, part two. *American Association for the Advancement of Science*. (www.sciencemag.org/careers/2000/01/abstract-killers-how-not-kill-grant-application-part-two) [last accessed 5 September 2017]

National Health and Medical Research Council (undated). Project Grants scheme-specific funding rules for funding commencing in 2018. Australian Government. (www.nhmrc.gov.au/book/nhmrc-funding-rules-2017/project-grants-scheme-specific-funding-rules-funding-commencing-2018). [last accessed 27 August 2017]

National Institutes of Health (undated). NIH Research Planning. (www.nih.gov/about-nih/nih-research-planning) [last accessed 5 September 2017]

Research Councils UK (undated). RCUK Strategic Priorities and Spending Plan 2016–20. (www.rcuk.ac.uk/documents/documents/strategicprioritiesandspendingplan2016/). [last accessed 27 August 2017]

ANSWERS TO ACTIVITIES

 READ–REFLECT–RESPOND 4.1

NATASHA'S ABSTRACT

1.　A concise, clearly written statement about the topic and its significance in the field (why it is important to conduct this study and what knowledge gap the study will fill).

Abstract: The abstract states that pregnancy is a life-changing and role-changing event that generates emotions, some of which may be psychologically disabling, particularly anxiety and fear. The disabling emotions can mitigate against a successful transition to motherhood and so it is important to investigate this so that women can be assisted in developing coping strategies.

Possible improvement: The abstract is concise in using 320 words. If it is known, then adding one or two facts about the proportion of women who experience these problems would make the abstract more hard hitting.

2.　Identifies the type of existing research on the topic; the methodological similarities and differences to your own study, and the methodological gap the study will fill.

Abstract: References of research relating to symptoms of pregnancy and the anxiety and fear experience are listed. All the studies reviewed have different research approaches, designs, samples, and data collection and analysis. The main conspicuous gap in the literature is the absence of research into women's experiences of anxiety and fear in the first trimester.

Possible improvement: A very brief naming of the discussions and debates in the prior research would add factual information to the abstract. A summary sentence also about the actual variety of research designs used in other studies would add further information and, more explicitly, make the point about why this is an issue.

3.　Describes the study in terms of aims and objectives, research approach and design in order to show how the gaps and omissions will be addressed.

Abstract: The aim of the study is to explore women's experiences of anxiety and fear in the first trimester of pregnancy. The means of obtaining the information are in-depth interviews and the administration of a questionnaire. A grounded theory approach will be used to collect and analyse the data of the interviews. The timing of the investigation, first trimester, will accommodate the major omission in previous studies and add new knowledge about the emotions experienced during this trimester.

Possible improvement: None suggested.

4.   States what significant outcomes the study will achieve.

Abstract: Once identified, an education programme can be introduced to assist women to learn coping strategies.

Possible improvement: None suggested.

LIANG'S ABSTRACT

1.   A concise clearly written statement about the topic and its significance in the field (why it is important to conduct this study and what knowledge gap the study will fill).

Abstract: Depression, diabetes and heart disease are the leading disease burdens in Australia being identified as National Health Priority Areas. Coronary heart disease (CHD) and diabetes frequently co-exist and the impact of depression on both conditions has been shown to result in significantly worse mortality and morbidity, as well as increases in health care costs. These chronic conditions are managed in the main in General Practice, and it is in this setting the majority of patients seek help, however GPs have limited time to manage the complex care needs of their patients.

Possible improvement: The abstract is concise in using 338 words. If it is known, adding one or two facts about the proportion of the population who experience the problems would make the abstract more hard hitting.

2.   Identifies the type of existing research on the topic; the methodological similarities and differences to your own study, and the methodological gap the study will fill.

Abstract: The international literature has shown that chronic illness care benefits from comprehensive and multifaceted health service delivery, and that General Practices are central to the success of coordinated chronic disease management.

Possible improvement: No detail is summarized about previous studies and so it cannot be seen what method gap this study is addressing.

3.   Describes the study in terms of aims and objectives, research approach and design in order to show how the gaps and omissions will be addressed.

Abstract The research aims are to (1) develop and test a training programme for general practitioners and practice nurses in the screening, assessment and management of depression in patients with heart disease and/or diabetes; and (2) to test the feasibility of practice nurses screening, assessing, collecting data, counselling, referring, reviewing and monitoring patients with co-morbid depression, and heart disease and/or diabetes. The design is a cluster-randomized intervention trial that will recruit 18 General Practices in order to generate 450 patients, with physiological, psychological and lifestyle measures taken at 3, 6 and 12 months. The primary clinical outcome will be a change in depression scores.

Possible improvement: As the previous study methods are not mentioned, how the gap is being addressed is not clear.

4.   States what significant outcomes the study will achieve.

<u>Abstract</u>: This project will lead to a tested model for assessment and treatment of co-morbid depression and heart disease and/or diabetes that is based both on sound research findings and the way that Australian General Practice is developing. The study will set up systems within General Practices to demonstrate how the care of co-morbid depression and heart disease and/or diabetes can be funded successfully using the new Medicare Benefits Schedule Item Numbers.

<u>Possible improvement</u>: The anticipated specific benefit outcome for patients and General Practice staff could be stated.

READ-REFLECT-RESPOND 4.2
PART A – ASSESSING A TITLE

Title 1: The concepts are smoking and alcohol consumption and so the study problem and hence variables are named. The description of the study population is unclear as the number and location of the schools are not included. Specific information is needed about the nationality, ethnicity or spoken language of the students.

Title 2: The concepts are identified as music and dementia but the type of music is unclear. There is no information on the amount of music or the nature of the benefits. The residential status of the people with dementia is unspecified, as are their age, nationality and severity of dementia.

PART B – IMPROVING A TITLE

1.   An investigation into the dietary habits of Aboriginal and Torres Strait Islander peoples.

      Becomes:
      A survey of the dietary regime of Aboriginal and Torres Strait Islander children attending primary school in far north Queensland.

2.   Multi-measure pain assessment in women living with cancer.

      Becomes:
      Multi-measure pain assessment of elderly Canadian women living with cancer in aged care facilities in Toronto.

3.   Culturally-based health care practices of Zulus.

      Becomes:
      A mixed methods exploration of culturally-based health care practices of Zulu men living in compounds in South Africa.

4.   The experiences of postnatal women's use of telemedicine.

      Becomes:
      The self-reported experiences of early postnatal Chinese women's use of telemedicine.

5.   An exploration of the experiences of Cultural Safety Educators overseas.

      Becomes:
      A qualitative study exploring the experiences of Cultural Safety Educators in rural communities in the Philippines.

READ–REFLECT–RESPOND 4.4

CULLING WORDS IN NATASHA'S ABSTRACT

Pregnancy is life- and role-changing for a woman, and can generate feelings of bewilderment, joy, amazement, confusion, anxiety, fear and ambivalence. Physical changes, over which the woman has little control, cause discomfort; the woman often becomes emotionally labile, and may experience vagueness and memory impairment. Of significance to the woman is anxiety and fear of the unknown.

Physical, emotional and cognitive symptoms of pregnancy are widely debated in the literature (Byrne et al., 2014; Darwin et al., 2015; Davis-Floyd, 1992; Gross and Pattison, 1995; Hall et al., 2009; Harvey, 1992; LeBlanc, 1999; Lewellyn-Jones, 1998; Schneider, 2002; Usher, 1990); however, exploring anxiety and fear in the first trimester has not been addressed. This is a stark omission. Experiences of anxiety and fear need to be investigated to assist women in developing coping strategies. The studies reviewed have different research approaches, samples, times at which questionnaires or interviews are administered, and data collection and analysis strategies.

First-time pregnant women, attending an antenatal clinic, in their first trimester will be invited to participate in a one hour in-depth interview in their home as well as completing the 'Ways of Coping Questionnaire (WCQ)', a self-report questionnaire (Folkman and Lazarus, 1988). Grounded theory will guide data collection and analyses.

The findings could inform the design of an intervention programme to instil confidence about situations that produce anxiety and fear, e.g. an app for communication between a woman, her partner, and clinic staff or group sessions of Mindfulness Based Childbirth Education (MBCE).

249 words

ANSWERS TO ACTIVITIES

REVISION

1. F
2. T
3. T
4. F
5. T

STEP FIVE

FEASIBILITY, TRACK RECORD AND TEAMS

CONTENT

Feasibilty

Track record and capability based on research opportunity

Putting together a research team

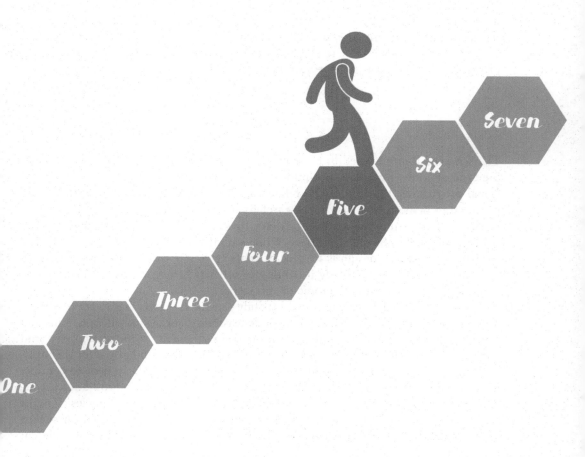

KEY TERMS/CONCEPTS

- Practicability of study design
- Institutional environment
- Team expertise
- Track record – Research Opportunity and Performance Evidence
- Early career researcher

INTRODUCTION

The research that you are proposing may well be dealing with an important problem, and you may have a rigorous research design and the anticipated outcomes may be significant, but are you able to show the committee that the research can be done with the resources available and given your capabilities? In other words you need to show the committee through your proposal that the study is feasible. The committee may well be impressed by an important study, but if they cannot see that you can conduct the study, they are not likely to approve it.

There are two broad aspects that a committee will consider under feasibility. First, can the study as proposed actually be conducted – is it feasible? And second, do the researcher and research team have a track record to show that they have research capabilities and can deliver research outcomes – can they do it? Finally, a committee might also want to see how the conduct of the proposed research will provide experiences for junior researchers and so build their future capacity.

FEASIBILITY

The term feasibility is used in research in two related contexts. The first relates to the type of study, for example a pilot study is a feasibility study to test the operational procedures; the second and related application refers to what is written in a proposal to demonstrate that the researchers have the skills, capacity and resources to ensure that a study can actually be done, that is, that it is doable, workable, practicable, and able to be put into effect. While a pilot study is one way to test whether a particular research design is feasible, it is also possible through the research proposal to demonstrate the likely feasibility of what is being proposed, and it is this second application that is the topic of this step.

There are many distinct aspects of feasibility of the research that relate to all sections of the proposal. These features include feasibility of the study design, aims and objectives, time, resources and institutional environment, team availability and experience, availability of the research site and participants, and also ethical considerations. For example, it is not likely to be feasible for one PhD student to conduct a ten country mixed methods study on the sexual behaviour of 3000 adolescents, comparing those born in European, Middle Eastern and Asian countries. First, it would be difficult to design such a large study across cultural groups on such a sensitive topic. Second, the project would be larger than a PhD and so one student is not likely to have the skills, resources or time that such a project would need. And third, it is unlikely that a PhD student could put together and lead a team needed for a complex project that requires highly experienced research leadership.

No matter how significant a contribution you believe your study will make (see the previous step), there is no point in pursuing a study if it is not feasible, that is, if there are impediments to its successful conduct. We will now explain each one of the different aspects of feasibility.

STUDY DESIGN – CAN IT BE DONE?

A committee will want to be assured that a study is achievable. This overall assessment of feasibility relates to the practicability of a research design. For instance, it would not be possible, at least ethically, to conduct a randomized controlled trial to test whether smoking caused lung cancer, as it would not be permissible to randomly administer a potentially dangerous intervention to one group of study participants. However, a cohort study, where one or more samples are followed prospectively, could actually be conducted on those who are smokers and those who are not. Another example could be of a researcher wanting to video labouring women's facial expressions during contractions in order to find out if there are cultural differences in response to pain. The hospital research committee may refuse permission if they consider this activity to be an intrusion of privacy and a disturbance of hospital routine.

Similarly, research on sensitive topics such as sexuality require careful consideration related to participant recruitment in the study design in order for it to be practically possible, as many people may have reservations about taking part in a study on such a topic. In these cases a study may not be feasible because a sample of participants cannot be obtained. It is often difficult to recruit a sufficient sample for studies that seek to involve GPs and, unless a researcher has sufficient credibility and influence, then a study may not be feasible.

Feasibility of the study design also includes the technical skills required, the researchers' own availability and time (e.g. release from other commitments), the duration of time needed to complete the study (e.g. the ability to maintain participants through a long study), financial resources available (e.g. the budget), access to the research site and participants, and the capability to use rigorous data collection tools and analysis. Often researchers will conduct a pilot study to test all of these aspects of the study design to see if they are feasible. If all of these aspects do not fit together in what looks like a feasible study then the committee may refuse approval, or at best send the proposal back with questions for clarification.

AIMS AND OBJECTIVES

The aim of the research identifies the research problem and should be feasible. There would be no point in developing a research project and submitting it to a research committee or funding agency if the researchers had any doubt that the aims and objectives of the study were not achievable. The aims constitute the boundaries of the research and prescribe the purpose of the study. They should therefore be specific, clear, focused on the research problem and succinct. Clarity when thinking about the aims is very important because what you decide regarding the aims will guide your literature search and the design of your study (methodology, venue, participants, inclusion/exclusion criteria, data collection and data analysis). The aims and objectives need to be feasible and within the research capacity of the proposer.

For example, on the topic of injuries in the workplace, an aim could be 'to investigate the extent, nature and outcome of the workplace injuries in a major automotive plant over a 12 month period'. Objectives specify the outcomes and are the more detailed statements about what research will be conducted, and specifically, how the aim will be achieved. Appropriate objectives for this aim could be the following:

1. To establish the incidence and cause of documented injuries through the workplace injury reporting system.
2. To determine diagnosis and treatment as documented in the workplace First Aid Station notes.
3. To establish return to work and rehabilitation outcomes as documented in injured worker employment files.

At face value the aim and objectives logically fit and the study required to achieve the objectives would be feasible, however, for this, the researcher would need to show that they have the required background, skills, resources, and access to the workplace and the related records.

TOP TIP

Objectives are subsidiary to aims and describe how the aims are to be achieved.

TIME

The time frame over which you have designed your study needs to be realistic. Some members on the review committee will be experienced researchers and they will know how long studies can take, such as the time taken in obtaining permission to access a research site; time taken to build a cohesive research team; time taken to recruit participants to the study; time taken to travel to collect data and analysis, and so on. New and inexperienced researchers can underestimate the time factor and should be guided by more experienced researchers on the team or their supervisors.

Time is also a factor in terms of how much time you and others are able to commit to the research study. If you are currently employed and have teaching commitments, you need to account for how much time you are realistically able to put aside to conduct the proposed study. It is also relevant to consider how ambitious your proposed study is in relation to other life commitments, such as to your family.

The time to manage the research team and the time to gain access to the research site and participants need to be assessed and to account for differences if the research were to be conducted on one site or spread over many sites, and if extensive time were required in the field. Time must also be allocated for the dissemination of your research outcomes at conferences, in writing the report, and in writing journal papers. If your study is for a higher degree you need to establish if appropriate and qualified supervision is available within your time frame, as you do not want a supervisor to leave half way through your Masters or PhD.

RESOURCES AND INSTITUTIONAL ENVIRONMENT

Regardless of whether you will apply for funding from a grant agency or a scholarship, and even if you have no external funds, a statement of resources is required to be submitted with the proposal. For instance, if you are on the staff at a university or enrolling in a research degree, you may enjoy certain privileges like office and computer facilities, copy paper and contact with your supervisor while you are working on your study.

A proposal will usually require a description of the resources available to assist the researcher and it is prudent to make yourself familiar with the types of support offered, for example interdepartmental assistance or external assistance with data analysis and use of laboratories. Students undertaking higher degrees should remember that guidance and support in writing a research proposal are also provided by their academic supervisor, and universities require that at least one supervisor, knowledgeable and competent in the student's topic area, is appointed for the duration of the study.

These 'in-kind' resources should be mentioned in your proposal, as well as any aspects that you might 'self-fund', for example, travel to the research site if this involves frequent and long trips. This shows the committee that you are aware of the resources needed to conduct the study.

The resource budget must conform to the requirement of *feasibility*, that is, whether costs have been carefully planned and will meet the study needs, be they for personnel or indirect costs. Each stage in the research should be linked, in a systematic way, to the budget. This will allow you to keep the overall feasibility of the project in mind and allow the review committee to follow your design and budgetary needs. If costs have been underestimated the study would not be considered feasible. More information on budgets is contained in Step 7.

Another resource factor is the environment of the research institution in which the researcher is based. A committee will be more inclined to approve a proposal if it comes from an established research institution, where there is a research culture that includes regular seminars and so on, and also a Research Office that can offer assistance with the management of a project. If you are working or studying in such an environment, the committee will see that you are surrounded by a culture that encourages research. Some proposal templates have a section that requires the researcher to describe this institutional context. For example, we recently reviewed a study that sought to examine the use of organizational change and that used participative research strategies to promote improvement in health policy. The researchers described how the Centre in which they were employed was located near to, and had longstanding links with, the National Health Service Executive. This proximity over time assured the committee that the Centre was a conducive environment for the conduct of this type of research.

TEAM AVAILABILITY AND EXPERIENCE – SUPERVISION

If your research idea is doable in terms of institutional support, it still needs an appropriate team with knowledge and experience of the topic available. We discuss putting together a research team more fully later in this chapter. If you are intending to conduct the research as the requirement for a higher degree (Master by Research or PhD), there needs to be appropriate supervision available.

AVAILABILITY OF THE RESEARCH SITE AND PARTICIPANTS

Unless data are to be collected from individuals either electronically or by post, it is necessary to ascertain the availability of the research site, be it a hospital ward, university classroom or field work in a health clinic. If data collection involves the recruitment of participants, ascertaining their availability should be considered in the early stages of your thinking. If you want to speak to people in a residential care facility or conduct an observational study, for example, it would be wise to speak to the Director of the facility about the research and the necessary procedures to be followed. There is little point in completing the design section of your proposal without knowing where and how your research data will be collected.

ETHICAL CONSIDERATIONS

In all forms of research, researcher integrity and honesty are of paramount importance. The content of your study relating to ethical principles is critical and should clearly demonstrate the ethical feasibility of your study and how you intend to address the ethical issues. This is dealt with in more detail in the next step.

READ-REFLECT-RESPOND 5.1

INSTITUTIONAL ENVIRONMENT AND SUPPORT

Many of the feasibility elements will be assessed by the committee from a reading across all sections of a research proposal; however, there may be a specific section in a template related to the institutional environment in which the proposed project will be located. Below is an example from Liang's proposal.

1. <u>Read and reflect</u>: Read this section and reflect on how Liang has provided information about the institutional context and the team expertise. Consider how Liang has built his team and who he has involved, how the roles are distributed and what will be involved in maintaining team contact throughout the project. Also consider how Liang has demonstrated the benefits that the team has achieved through previous collaboration.
2. <u>Respond</u>: Now respond with a section related to your own proposal about the supportive environment in which your proposed study will be conducted, and the availability and expertise of others on a team who will help you to conduct this research.

LIANG'S PROPOSAL SECTION ON THE INSTITUTIONAL ENVIRONMENT AND TEAM EXPERTISE

Research environment in administering and partner organizations

The research team at the Faculty of Health Sciences Mid Regional University come from the School of Nursing (Chief Investigators [CIs] Liang and Szabo), the Department of Public Health (CI McEvoy), and the Department of General Practice (Associate Investigator [AI] Davis). The Faculty of Health Sciences generated research income of $101M over the last three years, as the highest income earning faculty for the University. Within the Faculty, the School of Medicine had 92 PhD and 13 MPhil completions in the last 5 years. The School of Nursing had 23 PhD and 4 MPhil completions over the same period. The School of Nursing, in particular, employs three professorial positions with six related post-doctoral researchers in primary health care (including CIs Liang and Szabo), mental health, and aged care.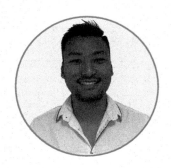

   AI Tonelli comes from the main partner organization, the Mid Regional Primary Health Care Service (MRPHCS). MRPHCS is the major provider of primary care services for more than 30,000 people in the region. MRPHCS run 18 clinics with 4000 annual referrals, 15,000 annual visits, and employs 150 staff. MRPHCS has a strong practice improvement culture promoted by a multidisciplinary Evaluation Unit that has undertaken more than 20 projects over the last 5 years.

Fit with strategic plan

This proposal addresses two of the nine goals in the Mid Regional University Strategic Plan. This is by engaging with stakeholders and local community through research with the MRPHCS (goal 1) and a focus upon research strengths at Mid Regional University in the area of health research (goal 5).

Role of personnel

Chief Investigator (CI) Dr Liang is a post-doctoral fellow in the School of Nursing. He has expertise in chronic disease management and in conducting practice-based research using both quantitative and qualitative methods. He will oversee the project, undertake data collection, oversee analysis, and contribute to the drafting of publications.

CI Dr Szabo is a statistician in the School of Nursing. She has expertise in statistical methodologies relating to a variety of quantitative designs in health services research. She will contribute to the development and application of the experimental design and to data analysis and the drafting of publications.

CI Prof McEvoy is research leader in the Department of Public Health. She has expertise in the use of research and evaluation in influencing policy and practice change specifically related to health care. She will contribute both to comparative data analysis and the development of policy change recommendations and strategy, and also provide mentorship to CI Liang.

AI Associate Professor Davis is a senior research fellow in the Department of General Practice. He has experience in the conduct of research in General Practice and will contribute to the recruitment of clinic sites and patients as well as to the development of the intervention programme.

AI Ms Tonelli is the MRPHCS Manager Strategy and Evaluation. She has academic status within the University. She will facilitate recruitment of participants through MRPHCS and provide advice about the implementation of the intervention and subsequent policy recommendations.

A research associate and research assistant will contribute towards implementing the intervention, data collection and analysis, drafting of publications, and maintenance of project records.

CIs Liang and McEvoy as well as AI Tonelli have previously worked together on Dr Liang's PhD project, and they have three joint publications from this work. CI Szabo has worked with CI McEvoy and AI Davis on numerous projects related to chronic disease management and they have authored five papers together on this topic.

The research team, chaired by CI Liang, will meet monthly via teleconference. CI Liang will meet weekly or more frequently as necessary with the research associate and research assistant.

TRACK RECORD AND CAPABILITY BASED ON RESEARCH OPPORTUNITY

'A track record statement is an argument demonstrating your capacity to carry out research and aims to convince assessors that you have the research skills, experience and ability to manage the project.' (Western Sydney University, undated). Addressing track record should include both a narrative statement as well as a CV that lists the achievements of all the CIs.

A review committee will want to know about you and your team, so that they can see the research projects and research outputs that the team members have conducted in the past. The committee may also want to consider your future potential should they approve your proposal. If you are a higher degree student then you are unlikely to have much of a research track record and your research team may well be just you and your supervisors.

Khoo (2012) says the following X-factor elements are what distinguish one application from another:

1. 'Excellent, existing relationships with relevant parties.' Present evidence of your past experiences of effective collaboration which have 'grown' your relationships.
2. 'Getting your research findings out there.' What were the results of your collaboration? What changes occurred in the field as a result of your findings? What opportunities arose through presentations at conferences? How will your team build on their particular research area?
3. 'Very shiny recognition by others.' Were the team and project recognized internationally as making a contribution to the area of research? Were any team members invited as keynote speakers? Was interest expressed in international collaboration in the research area as a result of networking?

Large nationally competitive research proposals such as those to the National Institutes of Health (USA), Medical Research Council (UK), and the Australian National Health and Medical Research Council (NHMRC), will need to provide a lot of information about researcher track record. Completing the track record section of these large grants can take a lot of time and effort, particularly if there are a number of chief investigators on the team who all need to have their track record described. The NHMRC allocates 25% weighting to track record when assessing project grants, and will want to know details about the individual team members, their influence in the field of the research proposed, and how the team will work together. While smaller grants will not require the same degree of detail, the following NHMRC (undated) descriptors give an idea of the kinds of information committees will be looking for.

Table 5.1   Australian NHMRC descriptors for assessment of team track record and capability

---

Research outputs relevant to the proposed field of research – includes most recent significant publications, publications that illustrate innovation and significance to past accomplishments, impact or outcome of previous research achievements, including effects on health care practices or policy, awards or honours in recognition of achievements.

Contribution to discipline or area – includes invitations to speak at international meetings, editorial appointments, specialist and high level health policy committee appointments.

Other research-related achievements – includes influence on clinical/health policy or practice or provision of influential advice to health authorities and government, impacts on health via the broad dissemination of research outcomes, e.g. via mainstream media, the community, or industry involvement.

Source: Drawn from the Australian NHMRC project grant rules for funding.

The following list can also be useful as a way of structuring the items to include for the track record of each research team member. Generally committees will only want this information for the named chief or principal investigators and not for the associate investigators:

- Peer reviewed publications – overall (highlight those in which you were the first author) and top 5 in the past 5 years (provide reasons for assessment of top).
- Research grants received (list investigator status, granting organization and amount).

- Contribution to the field of research (what your research has led to).
- Collaborators (list significant other researchers and research organizations relevant to this proposal that you have worked with).
- Community engagement (relevant to the topic of this proposal).
- Professional engagement (such as participation in your professional associations).
- International standing (invitations to international conferences, participation in committees, journal editorial roles, etc.).
- Supervision and mentoring of higher degree students.
- Participation in peer review (of journals and grant applications).
- Receipt of prizes and awards.

The track record of researchers needs to be considered against the opportunities that they have had to build a research career. Some proposal templates will have a section for this to be recorded if applicable. The Australian Research Council (2014: p1) defines this as a Research Opportunity and Performance Evidence (ROPE) Statement with the two elements described in the extract below:

> **Research Opportunity** is designed to provide assessors with an accurate appreciation of career history against a timeline of years since graduation from highest educational qualification. Assessors will recognize research opportunities and experience in the context of employment situations including those outside academia and the research component of employment conditions. Periods of unemployment, or any career interruptions for childbirth, carers' responsibilities, misadventure, or debilitating illness, will be taken into account. Access to research mentoring and other research support facilities and any other relevant aspects of career experience or opportunities for research will complete the considerations.
>
> **Performance Evidence** is designed to provide assessors with information that will enable them to contextualise research outputs relative to the opportunity of a participant. Both research output assessment and contextualising within disciplinary expectations of research impact are required. In addition to standard academic publications, research outputs can include grey literature, consultancy reports or reviews, patents and policy advice, competitive grants and other research support, higher degree student completions, major exhibitions, compositions or performances, plant breeding rights, registered designs, invited keynote and speaker addresses and other professional activities and contributions to the research field.
>
> (Australian Research Council, 2014: 1)

For those with a PhD, the number of years since gaining a research degree qualification will be relevant. A person recently awarded a PhD (generally up to 5 years post award) may be considered an early career researcher. The track record of an early career researcher is not expected to be extensive.

Someone writing a proposal for admission to a research higher degree may only have a small track record. In these instances the person's prior academic record will be important, particularly the awarding of Distinction or better grades in research-related topics, the receipt of any study-related awards, and evidence of any work-related activities that show critical thinking, problem solving, and writing skills.

- -

READ–REFLECT–RESPOND 5.2

ROPE STATEMENT

Below is an example from the ROPE sections of Liang's proposal, except for his listing of publications and grants. The example has been adapted from a real proposal with some fictionalization to retain anonymity.

1. <u>Read and reflect</u>: Read this statement and reflect on how Liang has provided information about his research opportunity and performance.
2. <u>Respond</u>: Now respond with a relevant section in your own proposal about your research opportunity and performance. If there is a template for your proposal, the sections may look a little different from those in Liang's template.

If there are other chief or principal investigators named on your proposal then ROPE information will be needed for them as well. As already mentioned, when the team involves a number of researchers, compiling this information can take considerable effort and time.

LIANG'S PROPOSAL SECTION ON ROPE

Details on career and opportunities for research over the last 5 years

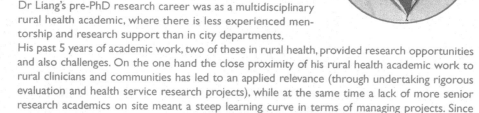

- It is 4 years since Dr Liang completed his PhD award in public health. Over the past 3 years he has been employed as a post-doctoral research fellow in the School of Nursing, Mid Regional University. During his part-time PhD studies he was also an evaluation project officer for 7 years in the Smith State University Department of Rural Health where he led a small team undertaking applied evaluation projects for regional health services.
- Dr Liang has had no career interruptions; however, much of Dr Liang's pre-PhD research career was as a multidisciplinary rural health academic, where there is less experienced mentorship and research support than in city departments.
- His past 5 years of academic work, two of these in rural health, provided research opportunities and also challenges. On the one hand the close proximity of his rural health academic work to rural clinicians and communities has led to an applied relevance (through undertaking rigorous evaluation and health service research projects), while at the same time a lack of more senior research academics on site meant a steep learning curve in terms of managing projects. Since joining the School of Nursing within the Faculty of Health Sciences his track record is developing an upward trajectory (see recent publications and grants listed in CV).
- Dr Liang has longstanding professional and academic relationships with Al Tonelli and also with the Department of Public Health, Mid Regional University (location of CI McEvoy) that were established in his rural health work and during his PhD. These relationships and his recent appointment to the position of post-doctoral fellow in the School of Nursing have enabled the timely development of this proposal. His location, now on a university main campus,

provides proximity to other public and primary health care theorists and methodologists. This has increased his capacity to develop a team-based research proposal on the impact of collaborative care on chronic condition health care. This capacity includes a greater focus on international scholarship, such as a recent travelling fellowship to Manchester University in the UK related to GP and nurse-led collaborative care. The fellowship built upon his PhD, and also prior work in rural health that involved evaluation of models to improve primary care for common chronic conditions.

Further evidence in relation to research impact and contributions to the field over the last 10 years

Policy advice

- Dr Liang's paper on 'Collaboration and local networks'(paper #5 in CV) provided a critical account of rural mental health planning. This was used in the Regional Mental Health Plan of rural Smith State as a way to optimize available skills and resources and thereby improve service access and acceptability.
- His work related to the role of agricultural support agents in mental health has been built into community structure and processes under the Smith State Farmers Association Mental Health Blue Print. This led to a broader social response to mental health servicing in the Health Department with the appointment of Drought Mental Health Liaison Officers (papers #8 & 9 in CV).
- His work on the development and sustainability of primary mental health care partnership to meet the needs of a rural Aboriginal population (paper #7 in CV) was used by the local partners and won a Mental Health Award from Smith State Department of Health. The framework that was developed has since been used by the Department in the roll out of its rural mental health service model.

Other professional activity

- Dr Liang is Deputy Editor of the Journal of Rural Health, and is on the editorial board of Open Community Health Sciences. He was one of the guest editors of the Rural Health edition of Rural Society. He regularly reviews for BMC Health Services Research, the Journal of Rural Health, Patient Education and Counselling, Australian Journal of Primary Health, Electronic Journal of Rural & Remote Health, and the Journal of Advanced Nursing.
- Dr Liang sits on the Community and Primary Health Care Faculty Advisory Committee of the Smith State Branch of the Public Health Association.

PUTTING TOGETHER A RESEARCH TEAM

As the assessment of track record will often involve consideration of the team, it is worth spending some time thinking about how you put a team together. Compared to a single investigator, a team of investigators will often be considered as more capable of conducting a study, particularly if the study is large, if access to study sites and participants is difficult, or if direct uptake of findings by stakeholders is a key selling point of the study. Hence, it is important to think about how the committee will assess the team that you have put together, the strengths of the team, and how it could further develop if the proposed research was approved and conducted. Five main considerations are (1) developing relationships that enable teams, (2) including end users on the team, (3) your position on the team relative to other members, (4) how to show team strength and development, and (5) managing a research team.

DEVELOPING RELATIONSHIPS THAT ENABLE TEAMS

To become a successful researcher it is important to network and build relationships with other researchers as well as with key people in the field of practice in which you have interests. These will be people within your own and other organizations, as well as people from the same and other locations (city or state) including other countries. When you have a personal relationship with others, they are more likely to help you out because they trust and respect you, particularly if you have been helpful to them in the past. They may feel an obligation to reciprocate.

Khoo (2011) makes the observation that '[its] not all about who you know, but if you don't know anyone (and they don't know you), then you're behind the eight ball'. This means that you need to put in the time to develop relationships early in your research career and to continue to develop these. It is ideal that this be commenced well before a research proposal needs to be submitted. Developing relationships can occur through attending the research seminars of others as well as giving your own, participating in conferences and also professional associations, or simply making contact with people who have similar research or practice interests to your own. Having a network of research and practice colleagues means that they can give you critique and guidance about your research ideas, they can help you to gain access to sites and participants, and also to translate your findings into changes to practice. When a research proposal needs to be written, you are then able to call on relevant people from your network to join your team.

INCLUDING END USERS ON THE TEAM

Grant committees will often look favourably on the inclusion of end users on a research team, often in the capacity as an Associate Investigator as Liang has done. By end user we mean patients, community members, clinicians, health service managers or policy makers, that is, those people who will have an interest in the research findings. An end user can provide advice and assistance on the conduct of the research, and also on the application of the findings. Choosing one or more end users for a research team requires careful consideration of the qualities, capacity and skills required of them, as you will have done when choosing other researchers to be on the team. You will want to make sure that an end user has a meaningful role and is seen by the other team members as a valued team member. If you want to include a patient as an end user member on your team, there may be a relevant patient organization, such as the Consumers Health Forum in Australia, you can approach to arrange for a patient to join your team, as people gained through these organizations often have the experience and confidence to take part in committee work and as a member of a research team.

YOUR POSITION ON THE TEAM

As you are the researcher who is initiating and writing the proposal, you are most likely to be the first named investigator. The main investigators are often called chief investigators (CI) or principal investigators (PI) and they will be listed as CI1, CI2 and so on. It is usual to list the CIs in the order of involvement on the project, that is, CI2 would be expected to be more involved than CI3. Others on the team who take a lesser role in the research are usually listed as associate investigators (AIs) or simply mentioned as staff in collaborating organizations somewhere in the proposal.

Committee assessment of the team will be focused mainly on the CIs and particularly the first named CI. As this is most likely to be you, it is important to consider your track record and whether you are ready for and have capacity to conduct the research that you are proposing.

There can be a temptation to include as CIs very experienced researchers, who have an extensive track record, just to make the team look good, rather than these members having a real role on the team. While it is a smart move to have senior experienced researchers on a team to assist more junior members, it is important that this role of mentor and guide also be included as part of a real role in the design and conduct of the study, including participation in the writing of papers. If you are a junior researcher proposing a project as CI1, say an early career researcher like Dr Liang, it is advisable to include an experienced researcher on your team, as Liang has done with Professor McEvoy as CI3.

As the first named investigator, the organization that you are affiliated with will be the administering organization to whom much of the benefits in doing the research will be attributed; these benefits may be research funds or simply prestige. If there are investigators on your team who come from other organizations (academic or practice) they may want to know what benefits they and their organization will receive by being on the team. These could simply be the reciprocal 'give and take' benefits described earlier, they may be the ability to use the findings to improve practice, or there may be some tangible interorganizational sharing of prestige and funds. If you are submitting your research proposal through a university, there will be a Research Officer who can provide advice about including investigators on the team who come from other organizations, and how benefits might be shared.

HOW TO SHOW TEAM STRENGTH AND DEVELOPMENT

Team strength and development will be determined by some or all of the following:

- Track record of the chief investigators, particularly the first CI.
- The role of each CI as described on the proposal and how these roles collectively bring the skills and expertise needed to conduct the project.
- The inclusion of associate investigators or organizational collaborators who bring resources to the project, such as links to the field to facilitate recruitment, and policy assistance to formulate actionable recommendations, etc.

- A description of how the research team will work together, including the role of each team member. A description of how team members have worked together in the past (if this has happened), and any outcomes, would provide some evidence to the committee of effective teamwork.
- How the team will provide opportunities for junior members of the team to be mentored and so gain the experience and skills needed to become more senior researchers. Team development can also include any opportunities that will be available for research degree students in the project. New researchers participating as members of a team would benefit by learning from established and high profile researchers' experience and they could use the occasion to also talk about their own research studies (e.g. Masters or PhD). From the perspective of the research team, postgraduate students and others can provide additional variety, energy and commitment to the project for having been given this opportunity.

MANAGING A RESEARCH TEAM

As the first named investigator you would take on the role as the team leader with the responsibility to manage the project. This will require personal leadership qualities and skills and a commitment of time from you.

Stanley and Anderson (2015) believe that an effective research team needs to have trust between members and a positive culture and that these occur when there is a clear agreed purpose, when members actively listen to each other, where they have a commitment to resolve issues and a strong sense of ownership of the team goals. They list the following six management tasks of the research leader:

- build trust and a positive team culture;
- clarify everyone's role;
- set the terms of reference and the agenda (team rules, expectations, team goals);
- hold regular meetings with minutes taken;
- celebrate success and reward contributions;
- manage project progress including budget and reporting.

If you are new to leading teams it would be useful to gain some training in the role. Often universities will run short courses in research leadership training so this will be worth looking into.

Finally, we should mention the possibility of conflict arising in the team and some suggestions for how to resolve conflict. Results from a qualitative study (Behfar et al., 2008: 170) suggest that groups who maintain or improve top performance over time share three resolution tendencies: '(1) focusing on the content of interpersonal interactions rather than delivery style; (2) explicitly discussing reasons behind any decision reached in accepting and distributing work assignments, and (3) assigning work to members who have the relevant task expertise rather than assigning by other common means such as volunteering, default, or convenience'. The leader of a research team should be attuned to conflict that may arise between members, and develop skills in dealing with conflict such as through leadership courses as mentioned previousiy.

Having read this section you should now realise that putting a team together takes effort. Getting your team together occurs during the proposal development stage where team ideas and roles are clarified and then, if the proposal is approved, in actually managing the project progress. The effort is needed well before a proposal is written. The time required to undertake this needs to be factored into your research development timeframe.

CONCLUSION

This chapter has covered Step Five – the step required in your proposal to show that the research you are proposing is feasible and that you and your team have the track record and capability to conduct the study. The amount of work required to complete this step (feasibility, track record and teams) in your proposal will vary according to the committee to whom the proposal is being submitted. For a PhD proposal, feasibility to conduct a study and hence what is needed to gain the degree will be a very serious consideration for a higher degree committee. Researcher track record will be an important consideration for a nationally competitive funding committee who will want to be sure that their investment is being made in a team who have a demonstrated track record and a team who are also building future research capacity.

The final two chapters of this Guide cover two main types of proposals: a proposal to an ethical review committee (Step Six) and a proposal to a grants committee (Step Seven).

REVISION

Below you will find five statements related to the content of this chapter. Indicate whether you think each statement to be true or false. The answers are given on p. 108.

1. Considerations about feasibility cover all aspects of a proposal.

    T/F

2. New and junior researchers can often underestimate the time needed to complete a study.

    T/F

3. If a very experienced researcher with a good track record is the first CI, it does not matter what organization the study will be based in.

    T/F

4. It is acceptable to be the first CI on a proposal as an early career researcher if the study is within your capabilities and if you have included experienced researchers on the team.

   T/F

5. It is a good idea to include an experienced researcher as a CI because they have a good track record, regardless of their real role on the research team.

   T/F

REFERENCES

Australian Research Council (2014) ARC Research Opportunity and Performance Evidence (ROPE) Statement. (www.arc.gov.au/arc-research-opportunity-and-performance-evidence-rope-statement). [last accessed 21 August 2017]

Behfar, K.J., Peterson R.S., Mannix, E.A. and Trochim, W.M.K. (2008) The critical role of conflict resolution in teams: a close look at the links between conflict type, conflict management strategies, and team outcomes. *Journal of Applied Psychology*, 93(1): 170–188.

Khoo, T. (2011) Networking and other academic hobbies. *The Research Whisperer*. (https://theresearchwhisperer.wordpress.com/2011/06/13/networking/#more-36). [last accessed 21 August 2017]

Khoo, T. (2012) How I assess a funding application: Part 1–Track records. *The Research Whisperer*. (https://theresearchwhisperer.wordpress.com/2012/05/15/assess-application-part-1/). [last accessed 21 August 2017]

National Health and Medical Research Council (undated). Project Grants scheme-specific funding rules for funding commencing in 2018. Australian Government. (www.nhmrc.gov.au/book/nhmrc-funding-rules-2017/project-grants-scheme-specific-funding-rules-funding-commencing-2018). [last accessed 21 August 2017]

Stanley, D. and Anderson, J. (2015) Advice for running a successful research team. *Nurse Researcher*, 23(2): 36–40.

Western Sydney University (undated). Track Record Statement. (www.westernsydney.edu.au/research/researchers/preparing_a_grant_application/track_record_statement). [last accessed 21 August 2017]

ADDITIONAL READING

Bammer, G. (2008) Enhancing research collaborations: three key management challenges. *Research Policy*, 37(5): 875–887.

Bennett L.M. and Gadlin, H. (2012) Collaboration and team science: from theory to practice. *Journal of Investigative Medicine*, 60(5): 768–775.

Burbules, N.C. and Rice, S. (1991) Dialogue across differences: continuing the conversation. *Harvard Educational Review*, 61: 393–416.

ANSWERS TO ACTIVITIES

REVISION

1. T
2. T
3. F
4. T
5. F

STEP SIX

WRITING AN ETHICS PROPOSAL

CONTENT

Ethical practice in research
Research ethics regulatory bodies

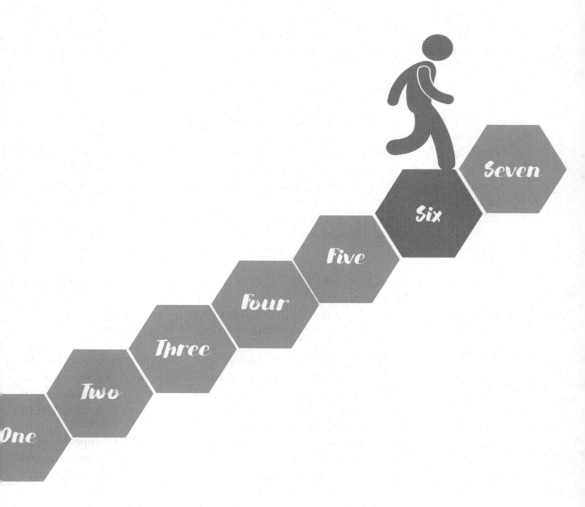

KEY TERMS/CONCEPTS

- Participant autonomy
- Informed consent
- Privacy
- Confidentiality
- Anonymity
- Risk/benefit
- Institutional ethics committee

INTRODUCTION

In most countries, research regulatory bodies require that research involving humans or animals should be approved by an institutional ethical review committee. A proposal to such a committee must describe the potential ethical issues that could arise in the conduct of the project and how these will be addressed should they occur. This is particularly important when the research is considered to involve 'high ethical risks' either because of the sensitivity or nature of the topic, the research design or the vulnerability of the study participants, which we will describe in more detail later in the chapter.

ETHICAL PRACTICE IN RESEARCH

Ethics is defined as 'The philosophical study of the moral value of human conduct and of the rules and principles that ought to govern it.' (Collins English Dictionary, 2006). Ethical conduct 'involves acting in the right spirit, out of an abiding respect and concern for one's fellow creatures ... with the sole intention to do good.' (Mandal Acharya and Parija, 2011: 2).

In relation to the conduct of research, ethical issues generally cover the following two areas:

- research practices that protect participants from injury, harm and discomfort, be they human or animal;
- research practices in the publishing of research to avoid plagiarism, providing misleading and inaccurate information, or withholding of information.

It is this first area that a researcher will consider when designing a study and about which an application to an institutional ethical review committee will be required. This is to ensure that what is being proposed meets the conventional standards for ethical research. Hence this chapter works through this first area to enable you to complete an application to an ethical review committee.

It is important to reflect on what constitutes ethical practices. Changes in what are considered ethical practices have occurred as a result of social and cultural mores, so what researchers considered appropriate or acceptable ethical practice in the past may not reflect current values. The Nuremberg Code of ethical principles was established in 1949 following the revelation that health professionals were engaged in unethical experiments on prisoners during World War II (Frewer, 2010). The Code was designed to guide ethical research practice involving humans in the future. However, these ethical principles were not always adhered to as some examples below illustrate.

There are numerous examples of past research that would now be considered unethical. We have provided below some examples that have involved false and coercive recruitment practice, concealment of the study purpose, and participation without being informed, and hence being unable to consent or to decline involvement in the research study.

For instance, the Tuskegee Syphilis study on African American men with syphilis, which began in 1932, recruited men on the understanding that they would receive free treatment for participating in the study; however, this did not occur. In the first instance the men were never told they had syphilis or that the researchers wanted to research the natural progression of the disease (Tolich and Davidson, 2011). The researchers can be considered to have acted unethically because they withheld important life-saving information from the men.

During the late 1950s and the 1970s, controversial medical experiments were carried out in the Willowbrook State Hospital in New York on intellectually disabled children. Hepatitis outbreaks were common at Willowbrook State School and in an attempt to discover how the virus was spread, 60 healthy children were fed live hepatitis virus. They became ill and died of the disease. The researchers can be considered to have acted unethically because of the coercion involved in recruitment, where admission to the hospital, and hence the provision of care, was made dependent on participation in the study (Reamer, 1998).

Milgram's experiments on participant obedience (Milgram, 1963) were motivated by events during the Holocaust. Milgram focused on the conflict between obedience to authority and conscience. He wanted to find out how far people would go in punishing others (inflicting pain) when told to do so by a person in a position of authority. The participants were initially told that the research was investigating the effect of punishment on learning; however, the real purpose was to examine obedience. The study involved a 'teacher' inflicting electric shocks on the 'learner' when they gave incorrect answers; the 'teachers' thought they were inflicting pain on the 'learners' and continued to do so under instruction from the researcher. The researchers can be considered to have acted unethically because they concealed the real purpose of the research from the participants, and also because the 'teachers' believed they were inflicting pain on the 'learners' and continued to do so.

The Cartwright Inquiry (1988) exposed a study conducted at the National Women's Hospital in New Zealand where women with major cervical abnormalities were followed. Coney and Bunkle (1987) reported that 948 women with precancerous carcinoma in situ of the cervix (CIS) and some with microinvasive cancer of the cervix or vaginal vault had, without their knowledge, received repeated diagnostic biopsies and cervical smears. Women with a positive smear were divided into two groups: those whose smear reverted to normal after 2 years, and those who, regardless of treatment, maintained a positive smear. This later group had been left untreated or undertreated in order to study the extent to which these lesions developed into invasive cancer. The women were not provided with treatment, had no choice in their selection, and they were not aware that they were being studied (Manning, 2009; McCredie et al., 2010).

Humphrey conducted a study called 'Tearoom Sex' intended to research stereotypes about homosexual men who participated in sexual acts in public restrooms. However, Humphrey initially concealed his identity and so there was no informed consent to be a participant in the study and the men were deceived about Humphrey's purpose (Nardi, 1995). In both cases the researchers can be considered to have acted unethically because the study was invasive and potentially damaging to participants; also, they were deceived about the nature of the study and were involved without their knowledge or consent.

The studies described above are considered covert, that is, when participants are unaware that research data are being collected; the researcher conceals from the participants the reason for their presence and withholds their true intentions. However, there are situations in which concealment may be necessary. For example, Bandura, Ross and Ross's (1961) Bobo doll study. Following the viewing of a model acting violently, the children were unknowingly observed as they played with toys. The purpose of the study was to measure the children's level of aggression. The researcher thought that the children would act more naturally if they were unaware of the purpose of the study.

Covert observation occurs in some anthropological studies where the researcher is *complete participant*, that is, where the researcher is accepted and immersed in the life of the group/community, and also when the researcher is *complete observer* – the researcher observes only and does not interact with participants.

TOP TIP

Giving informed consent to participate in a research study ensures the individual's autonomy and right to self-determination are respected.

There are also instances where the ethical procedures in a study are contested. For example, a two phase study on sexual assault and harassment in Australian universities in 2016 involved an open call for submissions to the Australian Human Rights Commission (AHRC) and an online survey with a randomly selected sample of current university students. The study was conducted on the understanding that the findings for individual universities would not be made public (Fileborn, 2017). However, the project faced intense criticism from student bodies and sexual assault activists about this decision. As a result, the universities agreed to make public the findings related to each university as a commitment of respect to the participants and also that the findings would lead to some action. This is an example where there is an ethical requirement that the cost of participation, such as the possible trauma of completing a survey on sexual assault, is likely to be less than the benefit that comes from the findings, such as actions to reduce future sexual assaults on campus.

Our final example as a Read-Reflect-Respond exercise below is different from the others we have discussed, but important when thinking about ethical issues in research team building (Step Five). Lee and Mitchell (2011) provide insights into their management of some sensitive and ethical issues, e.g. authorship, inclusion of another person in an ongoing project, student participation.

READ–REFLECT–RESPOND 6.1

Lee and Mitchell (2011: 463) discussed the ethical issues involved in having another person join an ongoing research project.

> With one of our current projects ... [we] judged that more data needed to be collected, analysed, and interpreted. Because the authors had many conflicting demands ... the study progressed far slower than expected...As a result, one of us suggested to the first author that another author might be added who would 'get things done'...Adding this person late in the process was necessary to complete the study.

The authors provide the following justification for the ethical issue in this situation:

> Had the new team member been added as a co-author only to finish minor editorial work (e.g. complete the references) and/or to 'pad' the team member's CV, an ethical question could legitimately arise over the sufficiency of contribution. A secondary issue might also be the adequacy of our role modelling for students. In the absence of a substantive contribution to the study, we believe that adding another co-author would have been wrong.

Hence the researchers indicated that the new invited author was expected to make a substantial written contribution.

Do you think that the authors' response to the potential ethical issue is adequate? Why?

ETHICAL PRINCIPLES FOR PARTICIPANTS IN HUMAN RESEARCH

The following are the general principles that should be followed in all research that involves human participants.

Participant autonomy

Potential participants must be free from coercion and any situations that may curtail their independence in the research study. This also extends to the way that potential participants are approached and invited to participate in the study. Some ethics committees do not approve of researchers approaching potential participants directly because of the concern that this may place them in an uncomfortable position if they wish to decline. While this can make recruitment difficult if it is required through some third party method, it is important that people are able to decline to participate without the researchers' knowledge and without any expectation on them or consequence as a result of their decision.

Autonomy also means an acknowledgement of, and respect for, the views and values of participants that may be different from those of the researchers and/or institutions conducting the research. Hence people who are invited to participate in a research study have a right to know exactly what part they will play in the study, their rights during the conduct of the study, the length of the study, assurance of confidentiality and anonymity, and their right to withdraw as autonomous individuals.

Voluntary participation

Potential study participants must be told in plain language that their participation is voluntary and that, should they not wish to participate, any treatment or intervention which may enhance their medical condition will not be withheld. Even if a participant, once enrolled, wishes to withdraw from a research project he/she must be able do so without prejudice.

Informed consent

Every participant in research must give voluntary informed consent to participate. 'Informed' consent implies that all procedures (interventions, timelines, risks, benefits) have been explained to the participant at his or her level of comprehension. In addition, the researcher should ensure, through questioning, that the participant has understood what his or her role is in the research project. A review of participants' understanding of information shows that participants may frequently not understand the information disclosed to them (Flory and Emanuel, 2004). Questioning every participant in a research study to confirm their understanding of process, procedures, and interventions is therefore important.

For a person to give informed consent they need to be of a legal age to give consent (the legal age may differ in different countries), and to be mentally competent to be able to do so having considered what the study involves and what is being asked of them. Factors affecting an individual's decision-making ability include dementia, mental illness or impairment, and learning disabilities. However, these conditions do not necessarily exclude an individual from making a decision. One should presume the possibility that individuals in these groups are able to consent unless professionally assessed and found incompetent. In this case, a person or guardian, who has the legal authority, may act on their behalf. Guidelines about age and competence are not always clear cut and can be open to interpretation, and hence an ethics committee would need to assess if parent or guardian consent was required.

Written consent

In addition to the verbal interaction between the researcher and participants described above (informed consent), there should be a record that includes an information sheet and a consent form, identical in content for both participant and researcher, to indicate how the research project was described in the verbal interview, and signed by the participant. In order to comply with ethical requirements, the consent form should indicate the following:

- "the signatory has received and read the information sheet or has had it read or explained to them;
- the purpose and structure of the project and his/her part in it has been explained and agreed with;
- any questions have been answered to the satisfaction of the signatory;
- the signatory understands that participation is voluntary and that he/she may withdraw at any time with no detriment;
- authority is given to consult a particular professional if required (for example, their general practitioner);
- a copy of the consent form has been received" (Denicolo and Becker, 2012: 71).

There may be some situations where a written consent will not be required, such as research with people who are illiterate, and in such cases consent may be recorded on a taped interview. A signed consent form may not be required on anonymous questionnaires where it is accepted that a return of the questionnaire signifies consent.

Privacy

This refers to maintaining the privacy of information, such as the details of a participant, and is an ethical and legal requirement in Australia (Privacy Amendment (Private Sector) Act 2000) (www.legislation.gov.au/Details). New Zealand has the Privacy Act 1993 (www.legislation.govt.nz/act/public/1993/0028/latest/whole.html). Privacy can be ensured through research practices that provide participant anonymity and confidentiality.

Confidentiality

Maintaining confidentiality means that any information given by participants is reported in such a way that information cannot be attributed to a particular individual. This means that the information given by individuals over the telephone, in writing, or during in-depth interviews, that could be attributed to them must remain private, protected, and in the safeguard of the researcher. If any information given by a participant that could be attributed to them is to be shared, then the participant must be informed, and agree to this in writing.

Confidentiality as regards participants themselves means that their identities and any information they provide will be concealed and safely stored. Caution should be exercised when assuring participants of confidentiality because, in some counties, data collection may be subject to Freedom of Information (FOI) legislation, or by subpoena, where the authorities are investigating a crime about which a study may hold important information. In Australia 'The FOI Act provides a right of access to documents held by Australian Government ministers and most agencies' (Australian Government, 1982, Freedom of Information Act).

Anonymity

Anonymity is provided by not recording the name or any other details that may identify a participant unless they agreed to this. In some studies, it may be required by an ethics committee that the identity of a participant not be known to the researcher, and this would mean that the researcher would not know who has participated and who has not, thereby making it difficult to follow up with non-respondents. This would be total participant anonymity. In other studies, the researcher may know who has participated and also which is each person's data, but use a variety of methods to ensure anonymity, such as giving the participant a number or a pseudonym so that they cannot be identified. In research studies where institutions, communities or locations might be identified by inference, it is important to ensure that appropriate safeguards are in place to prevent identification if they wish this. For instance, if the profession of participants are reported by their location, then in a small community of one doctor, it will be obvious who that participant is, even though they have not been named. A way to get around this is to group locations together where there are a small number of participants. As with people, some organizations may also not wish to be identified and so the practices for keeping the identity of organizations anonymous is the same as for individuals.

When using focus groups as a means of data collection then the identity of the group members will be known to each other, as well as the information that each member gives during the group. Although the researcher may not reveal the identity of group members in the written account, it cannot be guaranteed that group members will respect anonymity even though this may be set as a condition of participation. This needs to be made known to participants, then if they consent to take part in a group, they have done so in an informed manner.

READ-REFLECT-RESPOND 6.2

You are talking to your supervisor about your research design which involves interviewing 20 school girls in Year 12 about their alcohol consumption and smoking habits. What steps would you take to (a) determine whether the girls are competent to consent before seeking their permission to participate, and (b) identify potential ethical issues in this research project?

Participant protection - beneficence

Human beings must be protected from harm, both physical and psychological, that may result from participation in a research project. This principle is based on the right of participants to understand all information involving their participation in order to make an informed consent. Beneficence in research refers to doing good and protecting the participant against harm, physical or psychological. This includes the possible/potential consequences of participation. For example, if there are any risks involved in participation, such as the psychological risk in telling a researcher about past traumatic events, this needs to be made clear to participants. Therefore, any potential distress should be acknowledged and, if it occurs, suitable counselling provided.

Also in a research design such as a randomized controlled trial where participants are randomly allocated to a treatment (e.g. an intervention) or control group (e.g. placebo) without knowing to which group they have been assigned, they need to be informed about this, that even though they have agreed to participate, they may not receive the intervention.

Risk/benefit

The concept of risk/benefit refers to the probability of some future harm to those participating in a research study. A study presents minimal risk if 'the probability and magnitude of harm or discomfort anticipated in the research are not greater in and of themselves than those ordinarily encountered in daily life or during the performance of routine physical or psychological examinations or tests' (Oregon State University, undated).

Justice and respect

The ethical principal of justice refers to treating all participants fairly in all aspects of the study such as in the recruitment, participation burden, and in the benefits. The ethical principal of respect refers to treating the participant in a courteous manner, acknowledging their individuality and humanness, and behaving towards them appropriately.

READ–REFLECT–RESPOND 6.3

Data from the 2002/03 New Zealand Health Survey were used to assess the prevalence of self-reported experiences of racial discrimination in Maori (*n*=4108) and Europeans (*n*=6269) (Harris et al., 2006). Five questions were asked about: verbal attacks, physical attacks, unfair treatment by a health professional at work, or when buying or renting housing. Findings showed that both deprivation and experiences of perceived racial discrimination revealed inequalities in health outcomes between the two groups.

Exercise: You are planning to conduct a qualitative research study into racism in the health care system in New Zealand. You would like to interview 10 Maori health care professionals and 10 European health care professionals. Make a list of the issues that you would need to consider to observe the principles of participant privacy, anonymity, confidentiality, autonomy, protection, and respect for both groups.

RESEARCH ETHICS REGULATORY BODIES

Researchers undertaking research in any country should be apprised of the rules and regulations governing the particular procedures of the country in which they intend to undertake their research. In general, ethical conduct rules in research in the western world are based on those propounded in the Declaration of Helsinki in 1964 (World Medical Association, 2013). The United Nations Educational, Scientific, and Cultural Organization (UNESCO, 2005) continues their role of defining ethical conduct in research.

NATIONAL BODIES

Different countries have their own 'gold standards' for what constitutes ethical practice and ethical malpractice and these are made explicit in the policies of their respective national regulatory bodies.

In Australia, the National Health and Medical Research Council (NHMRC, 2003, 2015) provides research ethics review guidelines in accordance with the National Health and Medical Research Council Act 1992 as it relates to the whole community, to Aboriginal and Torres Strait Islander peoples, and also in relation to research involving animals. Compliance with the NHMRC National Statement is a prerequisite for those applying for NHMRC funding. The Animal Welfare Committee (AWC) in Australia advises NHMRC on issues relating to animal use for scientific purposes, and the NHMRC provides support and advice on animal ethical issues, including guidelines and information, to Animal Experimentation Ethics Committees (AEEC) and researchers (NHMRC, 2013).

In New Zealand, ethical conduct guidelines are published by the National Ethics Advisory Committee (2012) along with specific guidelines for research involving Maori and also Pacific Islander people (Health Research Council of New Zealand, 2010, 2014). In addition, in both Australia and New Zealand, guidelines are also produced for Disability Service consumers, children and indigenous groups.

In the USA, the Panel on Scientific Responsibility and the Conduct of Research (National Academy of Sciences, National Academy of Engineering and Institute of Medicine, 1992) oversee ethical issues. In the United Kingdom, the Academy for Healthcare Science has this role. In Canada, a tri-council policy (Canadian Institutes of Health Research, 2010) and also Health Canada and Public Health Agency of Canada (PHAC) (Research Ethics Board) formalizes the ethics review process and is responsible for overseeing and communicating to the Board on ethical research proposals (Health Canada and Public Health Agency of Canada, 2010).

TOP TIP

Even if your research study involves no living participants, consideration must be given to any people who may be affected by the publication of the findings.

INSTITUTIONAL ETHICS COMMITTEES

The procedures of various international ethics committees may differ but in general they are concerned with:

- promoting the rights of participants be they human or animal;
- ensuring the dignity, anonymity, confidentiality and privacy of participants;
- protecting the ethical environment for health care workers in health care agencies;
- providing advice and consultation;
- overseeing research ethics policies and procedures;
- reviewing research proposals involving human (Human Research Ethics Committee – HREC) and animal (Animal Experimentation Ethics Committee – AEEC) participants to ensure that ethical issues have been satisfactorily addressed.

In a reply to the question of why we have ethics committees, Aulisio and Arnold (2008) suggest 'that legal, regulatory, and professional forces drove the development of ethics committees, particularly as an alternative to litigation', and that the committees 'arose in response to a clinical need for a formal mechanism to address some of the value conflicts and uncertainties that arise in contemporary health-care settings' (2008: 417).

Membership

There are more than 200 HRECs in institutions and organizations in Australia. The composition of the ethics committees in Australia and the ethical principles and values to which the committees must adhere are determined by the National Statement on Ethical Conduct in Human Research (NHMRC, 2015). Membership of committees includes clinicians (doctors and nurses and other health professionals from all disciplines), chaplains, an ethicist from one of a variety of disciplines, and lay people.

Human research requiring ethical approval

Ethical regulatory mechanisms provide guidelines but have no legal force in Australia; however, most employers, funding bodies, journal publishers and research sites will require that a researcher has obtained an ethics committee approval. Trinity College Dublin has explicated the criteria for research ethics committees in accordance with the need for all their schools to have a research ethics approval policy in place. Not all universities, hospitals or academic institutions have two levels of ethics committees, but Trinity College Dublin (2014) does and it is worthwhile to provide a very brief account of their justification for two levels:

- Level 1 includes research not requiring ethics committee approval such as quality assurance studies, audits and research on publicly available information such as records, documents. The Committee chairperson's approval is required if there is an intention to publish.
- Research at Level 1 requiring approval by a Level 1 REC (Research Ethics Committee) includes: anonymous surveys; anonymous observation of people in public places; collection of non-invasive biological samples; interviews with non-vulnerable adults; action research; surveys where respondents can be identified.
- Research requiring approval by a Level 2 REC includes: surveys asking questions of a sensitive nature; questionnaires or observational studies involving vulnerable groups; projects involving a degree of deception; analysis of human tissue samples for which consent was not originally given; invasive procedures; vulnerable persons; research which may have legal, economic or social consequences for subjects; identification of illegal activity; payment to subjects and research that may potentially damage people or the environment.

Table 6.1   Categories to assess level of risk (Flinders University of South Australia)

Topic	Procedures involving	Participants
• parenting • sensitive personal issues • sensitive cultural issues • grief, death or serious/ traumatic loss • depression, mood states, anxiety • gambling • eating disorders • illicit drug taking • substance abuse • self-report of criminal behaviour • any other psychological disorder • suicide • gender identity • sexuality • race or ethnic identity • any disease or health problem • fertility • termination of pregnancy	• deception of participants • use of data or records from which individuals can be identified • covert observation • audio or visual recording without consent • recruitment via a third party or agency • withholding from one group specific treatments or methods or • learning, from which they may 'benefit' (e.g. medicine or teaching) • any psychological interventions or treatments • administration of physical stimulation (e.g. light treatment in eyes) • administration of devices to be swallowed (e.g. capsules) • infliction of pain • administration of ionising radiation • collecting bodily fluid	• suffering a psychological disorder • suffering a physical vulnerability • people highly dependent on medical care • minors (0–18 years) • minors (School of Psychology students aged 17) • people whose ability to give consent is impaired • resident of a custodial institution • unable to give free and informed consent because of difficulties in understanding information statement (e.g. language difficulties) • members of a socially identifiable group with special cultural or religious needs or political vulnerabilities • those in a dependent relationship with the researchers (e.g. student/ lecturer, doctor/patient, service provider/client, employer/ employee) • participants able to be identified in any final report or publication when specific consent for this has not been given • indigenous Australians

Source: Reproduced with permission from the Research Services Office at the University of Flinders, Australia.

An ethics committee will want the researcher to describe any risks and to balance these against the benefit that is anticipated from the research. In order to expedite ethical reviews some committees have a risk level checklist where low-risk studies are not subject to the full and lengthy committee deliberations of high risk studies. The categories used by the Flinders University Social and Behavioural Research Ethics Committee (SBREC) (undated) in South Australia to assess what are low risk or not are shown in Table 6.1. The committee chairperson will make a determination about the risk status of a research study and will not consider the study low risk if any of these features apply.

As more studies are being conducted, ethics committees are tending to require freedom for participants from any perceived coercion to the point that researchers may not be allowed to directly approach participants. Committees can also require that the researcher provide a very detailed written information sheet of the study that may be somewhat 'legalistic' and so frighten potential participants from participating. Hence it is worth putting effort into the participant information sheet so that it meets committee requirements, but is also inviting to potential participants (see later example of Natasha's participant information sheet).

CHECKLIST FOR YOUR INFORMED CONSENT STATEMENT

The following information should be included:

- title of agency (e.g. hospital, university, agency)
- invitation to participate
- basis for participation selection
- aim or purpose of the study
- an explanation of the rights of the participant, including what is expected of them, and that participation is voluntary
- sufficient information about the purpose/reason for the study
- a clear explanation of the procedures/interventions to be undertaken at an appropriate level of comprehension for the participant
- how to access treatment and compensation if injury occurs
- how to ask and where to address any questions or queries
- the duration, commencement, end and place of the study
- potential risks and benefits in participating in the study
- clarity regarding the confidentiality, anonymity and de-identification of the data of participants
- right of withdrawal without prejudice
- who has access to the data
- how the data are stored
- any conflicts of interest declared
- method of publication of results
- names and contact details of researchers, hospital, university, agency involved and ethics liaison office
- contact for further information or complaints.

As an example, Natasha's information sheet and consent form can be found in Appendix C at the end of this book.

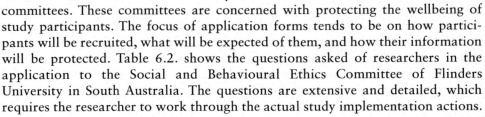

Ethics application form

As with research application forms, there will be some difference in the forms used by ethical review committees. These committees are concerned with protecting the wellbeing of study participants. The focus of application forms tends to be on how participants will be recruited, what will be expected of them, and how their information will be protected. Table 6.2. shows the questions asked of researchers in the application to the Social and Behavioural Ethics Committee of Flinders University in South Australia. The questions are extensive and detailed, which requires the researcher to work through the actual study implementation actions.

Table 6.2   Main topics covered in an application to the Social and Behavioural Ethics Committee (Flinders University of South Australia)

PROJECT DETAILS

Medical or health research involving the *Privacy Act*	• Will personal information be sought from the records of a Commonwealth agency? • Will health information be sought from a private sector organization or a health service provider funded by a State Department of Health?
Health research involving or impacting Aboriginal or Torres Strait Islander peoples	• Does your project comprise *health* research involving Aboriginal or Torres Strait Islander peoples?
Project information and data type	• How is the information to be sought – by questionnaire, interview, focus group, computer/online, experiment, secondary analysis of data? • Will participants be video or audio recorded, photographed or observed?
Research method	• *WHO will be recruited?* (e.g. students, staff, CEOs, children, members of public). • *SOURCE of participants* (e.g. organization, members of public, university, school). • *RESEARCH METHOD – what will participants be asked to do?* • *RECORDING – Audio/video recording/photographs.* • *WHERE will each component of the research be conducted?* (e.g. university, organization, private office, public).
Research objectives	• Briefly describe *how* the information which will be requested from participants addresses the research objectives.

PARTICIPANT INFORMATION

Identity and basis for recruitment	• Who will the participants be? • What is the basis for their recruitment to the study? • What component of the research will each participant group be involved in?
Participant numbers approached and population pool	• Please specify the number of people that will be approached (or an approximation if the exact number is unknown) AND the size of the population pool from which participants will be drawn. This is important for reviewers to know, especially if anonymity is being offered.
Source of participants	• From what source will participants be recruited (e.g. public, department, organization)? This provides information for reviewers about the possible vulnerability of potential participants.
Conflict of interest	• For *all* researchers, please indicate whether or not there is a conflict of interest. Please specify whether *any* of the researchers involved in the project have any role, or relation to, the source from which participants will be recruited (e.g. organization). Please indicate whether a possible conflict of interest may exist (financial or other interest or affiliation). For example; doctor/patient; employer/employee; lecturer/student; collegial relationship; recruitment of friends and/or family; other. If a possible conflict of interest may exist, please explain *how* this will be managed using an approach that will minimize any possible perceptions of obligation and/or pressure to participate.
Participant age	• Will any participants be less than 18 years of age? • IF YES, please indicate the age range of potential participants and confirm whether information has been presented in a manner and format appropriate to the age group of participants.
Informed consent	• Do participants have the ability to give informed consent? • If YES, please explain *how* participants will indicate willingness to be involved (e.g. completion of questionnaire, return of consent form, etc.). • If NOT, please explain why not. If participants will be aged under 18, indicate whether they will be given the opportunity to *assent* to research participation (e.g. sign parental consent form).
Cultural and/or religious background	• Indicate whether the participant group will be comprised of people from a specific cultural or religious background (for example, Aboriginal and/or Torres Strait Islander peoples, Greek people, etc.) OR if any such categories are likely to form a significant proportion of the population to be sampled.
Language	• Will there be any issues with language? If YES, please explain what the issues are and whether information will need to be presented in a language other than English. • Please also indicate whether anyone other than the researcher will be involved in translation of participant responses. If YES, explain how anonymity and confidentiality matters will be managed.
Contact and recruitment	• Please provide a *detailed* explanation of how potential participants will be contacted and recruited. For example, if making direct contact (e.g. face-to-face, in class, telephone) HOW will contact details be obtained and how will participants indicate their willingness to be involved in the project?

(Continued)

PARTICIPANT INFORMATION

Direct recruitment approaches
- Does recruitment involve a direct personal approach to potential participants (e.g. face-to-face, classroom, telephone) by the researchers or by other parties/organizations to be involved in contact and recruitment?

Information given to participants
- *What* information will be given to participants? For example, the letter of introduction, information sheet, consent form, survey, debriefing or feedback information. Please clearly outline *when* this information will be provided to potential participants.

Confidentiality and anonymity
- Indicate any confidentiality and anonymity assurances to be given to potential participants and explain the procedures for obtaining free and informed consent of participants *for each component of the research* (e.g. survey, interview, focus group, etc.).

Permissions
- Indicate any permissions that may need to be sought to conduct the research, recruit specific people, access existing data sets or post advertising material and attach correspondence requesting permission AND granting permission. If this correspondence is not yet available please respond that a copy will be submitted to SBREC on receipt. For example, permission may need to be sought from parents or guardians, teachers, school principals or the Department of Education and Children's Development. Recruiting employees may require permission from the organizational Head. Permission may also be required from data custodians, community organizations, etc.

Incidental people
- Indicate whether anyone may be incidentally involved in the research (e.g. members of the public, colleagues, family members, children, etc.). In certain professional studies consideration may need to be given to how such people will be informed about the research and how consent may be obtained for their incidental involvement. An oral statement given to a person/group incidentally involved *prior* to the commencement of the research may be sufficient.

Time commitment
- Indicate the expected time commitment(s) by participants AND the proposed location(s) for every component of the research (e.g. survey, interview, focus group, observation). This information should be clearly conveyed to potential participants in the Letter of Introduction and/or information sheet.

SPECIFIC ETHICAL MATTERS

Project value and benefits
- Outline the value and benefits of the project to the participants, the discipline, the community, etc.

Burdens and/or risks
- Notwithstanding the value and benefits of the project (listed above), outline any possible burdens and/or risks of the project for research participants, researchers and incidental people (e.g. possible identification, disclosure of illegal activity, transport of participants, conducting research in participants' homes, participant distress, etc.).
- IF any issues are raised, explain how the researcher will respond to each identified burden and/or risk.

SPECIFIC ETHICAL MATTERS

Concealment and debriefing	• Will the true purpose of the research be concealed from participants? • If YES, outline the rationale for, and provide details of, the concealment. • If YES, will participants be *debriefed* following project completion? • If YES, in what format will debriefing be provided? How will participants be informed of this process? (e.g. in the information sheet.)
Feedback	• Describe any feedback to be provided to participants that may be relevant to the research. • If YES, please (a) clarify how participants will be informed of this process; and (b) provide copies of any written feedback information to be provided to participants.
Questionnaires	• If participants will be required to complete a questionnaire, indicate what the arrangements will be for the secure and confidential return of questionnaires to the researcher (e.g. sealable self-addressed envelope, collection by researcher or someone other than researcher, secure collection box etc.). Please also indicate *how* participants will be informed of the arrangement (e.g. verbal instruction, information sheet, information listed at end of questionnaire, etc.).
Participant reimbursement	• Is it the intention of the researcher to reimburse participants? Refer to the Application Submission Guide available from the SBREC Guidelines, Forms and Templates web page for guidelines on participant reimbursement.
Data transcription	• Indicate whether data may need to be transcribed. If YES, please indicate who will transcribe the data (e.g. researcher(s), secretarial assistance, professional transcription company). If anyone other than the researcher(s) will transcribe data, confirm whether they will be asked to sign a confidentiality agreement, a template for which is available from the SBREC Guidelines, Forms and Templates web page.
Participant control of data	• Indicate whether participants will have any control in the immediate reporting and future use of data collected for the purposes of the research. Will participants have the ability to review and edit individual interview transcripts (if relevant) and/or the final report prior to publication? If YES, ensure that this is clearly explained to participants in the information sheet.

Source: Reproduced with permission from the Research Services Office at the University of Flinders, Australia.

 ACTIVITY 6.1   YOUR ETHICS
APPLICATION – STEP SIX

Using the list of questions in Table 6.2 as a guide, record what strategies you will use to ensure that your research is conducted in a way that meets the requirements of an ethical review committee.

CONCLUSION

This chapter has covered the ethical and legal issues involved in writing an ethics proposal, which is to gain the approval of an ethical review committee. While the completion of an ethics application can take some time because of the detail required, this will be worthwhile because you will then have a plan of each action required to recruit participants and how you will manage data collection. The focus of an ethics application is on how you will treat participants. The next chapter on writing a funding proposal moves back to a focus on the feasibility and benefit of a proposed study to meet the interests of the funding agency.

REVISION

Below you will find five statements related to the content of this chapter. Indicate whether you believe each statement to be true or false. The answers are given on p. 129.

1. Not all research on humans requires written consent.

   T/F

2. There are situations in research where deception is permitted.

   T/F

3. No researcher may involve a person in a research project without obtaining their informed consent.

   T/F

4. A researcher will sometimes be required to give information to third parties and so violate participant confidentiality.

   T/F

5. The main role of an institutional ethics committee is to protect the public.

   T/F

REFERENCES

Aulisio, M.P. and Arnold, R.M. (2008) Role of the ethics committee: helping to address value conflicts or uncertainties. *Chest*, 134(2): 417–424.

Australian Government (1982) Freedom of Information Act. (https:www.legislation. gov.au/Details/C2004A02562). [last accessed 08 November 2017]

Bandura, A., Ross, D. and Ross, S.A. (1961) Transmission of aggression through imitation of aggressive models. *Journal of abnormal and social psychology*, 63(3): 575–582.

Canadian Institutes of Health Research (2010) Tri-Council policy statement: ethical conduct for research involving humans [article 11.2]. Ottawa (ON): Canadian Institutes of Health Research, Natural Sciences and Engineering Research Council of Canada, Social Sciences and Humanities Research Council of Canada.

Cartwright, S.R. (1988) *The report of the committee of inquiry into allegations concerning the treatment of cervical cancer at National Women's Hospital and into other related matters*. Auckland, New Zealand: Government Printing Office.

Collins English Dictionary (2006) 8th edn. Glasgow: Harper Collins.

Coney, S. and Bunkle, P. (1987) "An Unfortunate Experiment at National Women's". *Metro Magazine*, Auckland, New Zealand pp 47–65.

Denicolo, P. and Becker, L. (2012) *Developing Research Proposals*. London: SAGE Publications.

Fileborn, B. (2017) How ethical is sexual assault research? (https://theconversation.com/how-ethical-is-sexual-assault-research-75768?). [last accessed 22 August 2017]

Flinders University: Social and Behavioural Research Ethics Committee (undated) Low or Negligible Risk Assessment. Flinders University. (www.flinders.edu.au/research/researcher-support/ebi/human-ethics/resources/forms.cfm). [last accessed 1 December 2017].

Flory, J. and Emanuel, E. (2004) Interventions to improve research participants' understanding in informed consent for research: a systematic review. *JAMA*, 292(3): 1593–1601.

Frewer, A. (2010) Human rights from the Nuremberg Doctors Trial to the Geneva Declaration. Persons and institutions in medical ethics and history. *Medicine, Health Care and Philosophy*, 13(3): 259–68.

Harris, R., Tobias, M., Waldegrave, K., Karlsen, S. and Nazroo, J. (2006) Effects of self-reported racial discrimination and deprivation on Maori health and inequalities in New Zealand: cross-sectional study. *Lancet*, 367(9527): 2005–2009.

Health Canada and Public Health Agency of Canada (PHAC) REB (Research Ethics Board) (2010). (www.canada.ca/en/health-system-services/health-canada-public.../) [accessed 26 November 2017]).

Health Research Council (HRC) of New Zealand (2010) Te Ara Tika: Guidelines for Maori Research Ethics. (www.hrc.govt.nz/news-and-publications/publications/te-ara-tika-guidelines-m%C4%81ori-research-ethics-framework-researcher). [last accessed 5 September 2017]

Health Research Council (HRC) of New Zealand (2014) Guidelines on Pacific Health Research. (www.hrc.govt.nz/sites/default/files/Pacific%20Health%20Research%20Guidelines%202014.pdf). [last accessed 5 September 2017]

Lee T.W. and Mitchell, T.R. (2011) Working in research teams: lessons from personal experiences. *Management and Organization Review*, 7(3): 461–469.

Mandal, J., Acharya, S. and Parija, S.C. (2011) Ethics in human research. *Tropical Parasitology*, 1(1): 2–3.

Manning, J. (ed.) (2009) *The Cartwright Papers: Essays on the Cervical Cancer Inquiry, 1987–88*. Wellington, NZ: Bridget Williams Books.

McCredie, M.R., Paul, C., Sharples, K.J., Baranyai, J., Medley, G., Skegg, D.C. and Jones, R.W. (2010) Consequences in women of participating in a study of the natural history of cervical intraepithelial neoplasia 3. *Australian and New Zealand Journal of Obstetrics and Gynaecology*, 50(4): 363–370.

Milgram, S. (1963) Behavioral study of obedience. *Journal of Abnormal and Social Psychology,* 67(4): 371–378.

Nardi, P.M. (1995) "The Breastplate of Righteousness". Twenty-five years after Laud Humphreys' Tearoom Trade: impersonal sex in public places. *Journal of Homosexuality,* 30(2): 1–10.

National Academy of Sciences, National Academy of Engineering and Institute of Medicine (1992). Panel of Scientific Responsibility and the Conduct of Research. *Responsible Science: Ensuring the Integrity of the Research Process: Volume 1.* Washington (DC): National Academies Press (US).

National Ethics Advisory Committee (2012) Streamlined ethical guidelines for health and disability research. (http://neac.health.govt.nz/streamlined-ethical-guidelines-health-and-disability-research). [last accessed 21 August 2017]

National Health and Medical Research Council (NHMRC) (2003) Values and Ethics – Guidelines for Ethical conduct in Aboriginal and Torres Strait Islander Health Research. Canberra, Australia.

National Health and Medical Research Council (NHMRC) (2013) Australian code for the care and use of animals for scientific purposes 8th edn. Canberra, Australia.

National Health and Medical Research Council (NHMRC) (2015) National Statement on Ethical Conduct in Human Research. Canberra, Australia. (www.nhmrc.gov.au/health-ethics/human-research-ethics-committees-hrecs/human-research-ethics-hrecs/national). [last accessed 21 August 2017]

Oregon State University (undated) (https://oregonstateducation/academics [accessed 26 November 2017]).

Reamer, F. (1998) *Social work research and evaluation skills.* New York: Columbia University Press.

Tolich, M. and Davidson, C. (2011) *Getting Started. An introduction to research methods.* Auckland, New Zealand: Pearson Education.

Trinity College Dublin (2014) Criteria for Research Ethics Committees. (www.tcd.ie/medicine/asseets/pdf/Criteria-for-Research-Ethics-Committees-Final.pdf). [accessed 29 November 2017]

UK Academy for Healthcare Science. (www.ahcs.ac.uk). [last accessed 5 July 2017]

UNESCO Universal Declaration on Bioethics and Human Rights. 2005. (www.unesco.org/new/en/social-and-human.../bioethics/bioethics-and-human-rights/).

World Medical Association (2013) Declaration of Helsinki: Ethical principles for medical research involving human subjects. *JAMA,* 301(20): 2191–2194.

ANSWERS TO ACTIVITIES

 READ–REFLECT–RESPOND 6.2

Assessing competency to participate in a research study is to ensure the participant understands clearly what is required of him/her:

Each student will be given the information sheet to read. In order to ensure that the information has been understood, ask the student some questions like:

1. I'm looking for students who either drink alcohol or smoke. Do you drink alcohol or smoke?
2. Tell me what information you think I want from you in this study.
3. How do you think I want to get your responses? (e.g. questionnaire, face-to-face interview, focus group).
4. How will I keep your name and information confidential?
5. What are the risks to you in this study?
6. What benefits to you are there for your participation in this study?

- -

REVISION

1   T
2   F
3   T
4   T
5   T

STEP SEVEN

WRITING A FUNDING PROPOSAL

CONTENT

- Planning ahead
- Working with timelines
- Guidelines and form fillers
- Strategic budgeting
- Appendices, letters of support
- Committee processes

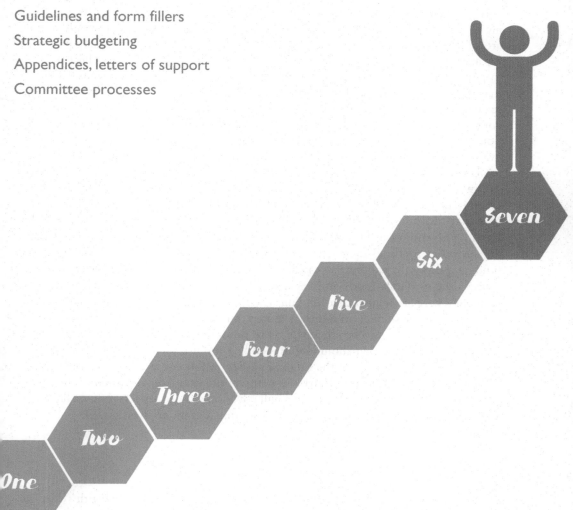

KEY TERMS/CONCEPTS

- Early career researcher
- Grants calendar
- Research support office
- Seeding grant
- Large competitive grant
- Form filler
- Gantt Chart
- Rejoinder

INTRODUCTION

If you engage in research beyond a PhD you will almost certainly be involved in writing a grant proposal to seek the funds that are needed to conduct your study. If you are a higher degree research student then you may also be writing a funding proposal for a scholarship for your living expenses, to cover field expenses to collect data or to pay for costs of analysis. A grant proposal is different from the proposal writing that we have so far covered in the previous chapters, where the goal is to convince a review committee that your research is worthwhile, that the design is sound, is within your capabilities, and is ethical. A funding proposal is all of these things, but in addition it will be competing against other proposals for the limited funds that are available. In the national competitive grant schemes in Australia and New Zealand, the USA, the UK and in Europe, success rate in the most prestigious schemes can be as low as 15% with grant templates often being between 100 to 150 pages. These schemes include the National Health and Medical Research Council (Australia), the National Institutes of Health (USA), the Medical Research Council (UK), and the Canadian Institutes of Health Research (CIHR). For this reason, submitting a funding proposal to these schemes needs to stand out from the crowd. Many good funding proposals will not be awarded because the number of applications far exceeds the available funds and because the criteria for acceptance will be set at a high bar. There are many other funding schemes where the competition is not as great and are often for smaller amounts of money, but you will still be competing against other applications. So to be successful, your funding proposal needs to be distinctive and stand out as one that should be funded because it is an exceptionally good proposal, it meets the criteria of the funding agency, and because it is value for money.

Writing a funding proposal involves many of the same steps covered in the previous chapters and so in this chapter we will cover only those aspects that we have not already covered and that are particular to writing a grant application.

PLANNING AHEAD

If you were to write an application to the National Institutes for Health (USA) as your first funding application you would not be making a good investment of your time as you would almost certainly fail. In fact, you would probably struggle to write the application as a novice without having some experience in seeking research grants. For this reason it is wise to plan your research funding strategies over a long period, where you seek funding in stages. The first application could be for a small grant that gets you started, possibly an internal scheme in your own organization, then moving onto larger grants over time that build on your outcomes and past grant success. Some grant schemes set aside funding applications for novice researchers, called early career researchers (ECR) in Australia, who have been awarded their PhD in the last 5 years.

While you should aim for a grant that will give you a reasonable chance of success, it can be a strategic move at times to also submit an application to a scheme that is a step higher than what you consider will be achievable. You do this in order to get the experience of writing such a grant and also to get feedback on what you could improve (if the scheme does provide reviewer feedback).

SEARCHING FOR GRANT SCHEMES

If you are in a university there will probably be a 'grants bulletin' that is circulated. An example from one our own universities (Flinders) is the 'Flinders University Research Services Office: Grants Bulletin', which is produced monthly. The bulletin lists current opportunities by the broad discipline area (social sciences, health, engineering, etc.), the grant scheme title and short description, a hyperlink to the grant scheme web page, and the internal and external closing date. For assistance you should consult the research office of your university or a similar support unit if you are located in a health service.

Other organizations also provide grant lists such as those from community and philanthropic schemes and, while these are often more focused on the implementation of activities to do good work (such as a welfare programme) or improve a service (such as a more accessible waiting room), they can also be a source of funds for research if there is evaluation or research associated with the activity. An internet search will reveal a range of these grant listing organizations, for example:

- Funding Central in the UK: www.fundingcentral.org.uk/default.aspx
- Grant Guru Community in Australia: http://community.grantready.com.au
- Grants Gov in the USA: www.grants.gov
- Grantwatch.com in the USA: www.grantwatch.com

A useful international resource that provides a worldwide database and search engine for the identification of research funding opportunities is 'Research Professional'. This can be accessed at the following URL: http://info.researchprofessional.com.

Many grant schemes are available on a regular cycle (usually annually) and so it is good planning to know what time of the year a scheme will be open. This enables you to plan ahead so that you can work to the timeline with a well prepared application. Most universities will also have a grant calendar that shows the annual cycle of major grant schemes.

TYPE OF GRANTS

Research funding grants fall broadly into three types – projects, programmes and fellowships – although they may be called different names, for instance a fellowship might also be called a scholarship.

A project grant is one where the purpose and focus of the application is to conduct one study. In this case the assessment of the application will be largely on the significance of the problem to be addressed, the rigour of the research design, and the capability of the research team to complete the study. In general most new researchers will apply for a project grant or a fellowship grant before applying for a programme grant.

A programme grant is an application for a larger amount of funds over a longer period in which to conduct a number of related studies that are needed to significantly advance knowledge and solve one or more problems. These are called programme grants because they are intended to cover a programme of work, are targeted at large teams of experienced researchers often across international teams, and involve industry collaborations. The assessment of programme grants focuses less on the rigour of individual studies (projects), and more on the innovation and strength of the research to solve a significant problem, the capacity of the research team members that will need to be at a high level often across multiple organizations and countries, and the level of partnership with organizations that will translate the research findings into solving the problem.

Research fellowship grants are designed to fund individuals as researchers over a designated time period. Fellowships can target very senior and experienced researchers, such as through senior and principal research fellowships, through to more junior researchers via post-doctoral fellowships and career development awards. These fellowships tend to cover all or part of the researcher's salary and some research infrastructure costs over periods of around 3 to 5 years. Fellowship grants assume that the researcher will seek other grants to cover the costs of running a research project or programme if this is needed.

In addition to these three broad grant types, where the funding sought is entirely through the granting organization, there are grants that require some proportion of the funding to be obtained elsewhere, most often from an industry partner. These schemes operate on a co-contribution arrangement so that eligibility to apply requires a proportion of actual funds to come from an industry partner, but with allowance for some in-kind contribution to be included, such as salaries, office costs, etc. The co-contribution grant schemes generally have a higher success rate than the wholly funded schemes and so, for researchers with good industry links, these grants can be a good option. In Australia, these schemes include the Linkage Grants provided by the Australian Research Council and the Partnership Projects Grants provided by the National Health and Medical Research Council.

In addition to the main health granting agencies that tend to fund biomedical research, such as the Medical Research Council (UK), National Institutes of Health (USA) and the National Health and Medical Research Council (Australia), there are schemes that focus on funding health services research, that is, on solving problems relating to the way that health services are organized and delivered. Examples include the following:

- National Institute for Health Research Health Services and Delivery Research (HS&DR) Programme that is funded through the UK National Health Service that can be accessed at the URL: www.nihr.ac.uk/funding-and-support/ funding-for-research-studies/funding-programmes/health-services-and-delivery-research.
- Robert Wood Johnson Foundation (USA) that can be accessed at the URL: www. rwjf.org/en.html.

For new researchers, or for researchers developing new areas of study, there are grant schemes that are generally small and that provide specifically targeted funds to get the researcher started. These might be called early career researcher grants, start up grants or seeding grants. They are generally easier to win than the grants listed above. With early career researcher grants it is wise to include more experienced researchers on the team as a co-investigator or mentor role, not as the first named chief investigator. These smaller grants work on the premise that a small amount of grant funds can be an investment that will, through the generation of some early data and publication, place a researcher in a better position to win a more competitive large grant.

 ## ACTIVITY 7.1 MAKE A LIST OF GRANT SCHEMES

Make a list of grant schemes that you consider will give you a likely chance of success given where you are at in your research career. You can do this by looking up your research office grants bulletin, consulting with your organization's research support officer and talking with research colleagues, or searching for a scheme on the internet. Your chance of success will be increased if your study is a topic or type of study that the scheme covers, and if your capability and track record are commensurate with the competitive level of the grant scheme.

WORKING WITH TIMELINES

Writing a grant takes time in order for it to have a chance of success. The time that is required should be clear to you by now, having worked through the various steps in this Guide. While there are stories of researchers working around the clock to get a grant application completed 'at the last minute', we have not actually met anyone who has done this successfully. Rather, we have sat on grant review committees where committee members have made disparaging remarks about poorly written applications that read as if they had been rushed because of mistakes, inconsistencies, untidy formatting, and so on. Submitting a rushed and hence poor application can create a negative impression and damage the reputation of the research team submitting the application.

Grant submission timelines can be known well beforehand, even before rounds are announced if these occur on a regular cycle. This means that a researcher can plan well ahead to ensure a well written application is completed by the submission date.

Included in this timeline should be the time for someone outside of the research team to read the application well before the submission date. This is to check, amongst other things, that it makes sense, that a compelling argument is made for the research with the proposed design, and that the credentials of the research team show that they are well equipped to conduct the study. Then there needs to be time for the researchers to refine the application based on any feedback. This means that the application needs to be sufficiently completed well before the submission date for this review and refinement to occur.

Grant proposals from a university will usually be submitted through the university research office, who will conduct a compliance check of the application to ensure that it meets all the eligibility requirements of the grant scheme. Research offices will set an internal submission date that might be a week or two before the external submission date (to the granting organization) in order to complete this check.

With required submission dates known, a strategic researcher will establish a timeline of activities that follow the steps in this Guide. This could involve many months of prior activity leading up to the submission date.

GUIDELINES AND FORM FILLERS

A researcher should write an application by following the guidelines of the grant scheme. An application is not likely to get funded if it does not meet the eligibility criteria for a grant, if it does not provide the information requested, and if it is not in the format required. While this would seem to be obvious, we have seen applications where this is not the case and so these applications are usually dismissed very early, sometimes before even reaching the review committee. Grant schemes generally have more applications than they can fund and so they first cull those that do not meet the guidelines.

Most schemes will have a specific application form or template, that is sometimes called a 'form filler' if it is to be completed online. Templates can be from a few pages for small grants to more than 100 pages for large grants. When completed online, form fillers can be notoriously difficult for unfamiliar applicants to work with, particularly if you want to include diagrams or special formatting. If the grant application is to be completed online then there is a chance that the grant website could crash and go offline at some stage in the writing of your application, so it is wise to familiarize yourself with the workings of the application template in the early stages of the proposal development and keep offline backups of your application. Many schemes will require that you register on their grants management system before you can commence inputting material on the form filler.

In Table 7.1 we provide an example of the size and information required in a form filler from the small grants scheme of the Faculty of Medicine, Nursing and Health Sciences at Flinders University.

Table 7.1   Sections in a template for a small grant

Scheme name	Seeding/Early Career Researcher Grants.
	Faculty of Medicine, Nursing and Health Sciences, Flinders University.
Purpose	Projects not yet suitable for competitive or external grant funding.
Eligibility	• Staff members of the Faculty of Medicine, Nursing and Health Sciences, Flinders University.
	• Early Career Researchers must be within 5 years FTE of receiving their PhD.
Funding items covered	• Direct research costs.
	• Minor equipment.
	• Project related travel.
	NOTE:
	Salary contributions not to be used for backfilling existing positions. Maximum funding $AUD 20,000 over 18 months.
Assessment criteria	60% – Scientific quality.
	20% – Strategic intent and focus (how the grant will assist applicants make further application for an external grant).
	20% – Track record of all chief investigators over the past 3 years.

APPLICATION

Cover page (1 page)	• Application title.
	• Significance/media ready/lay description (2000 characters max).
	• ERA 4 digit Field of Research (FoR) code (Australian coding used to classify the field/topic of the research).
	• Early career status.
Chief investigator details (1 page per investigator up to 10 chief investigators)	• Identifying and contact details.
	• Career disruptions (such as pregnancy, caring responsibilities, illness).
	• Publications (last 3 years).
	• Patents (last 3 years).
	• Time commitment to project (hours per week).
Associate investigator details (1 page per investigator, up to 10 associate investigators)	• Identifying and contact details.
	• Employing institution.
	• Time commitment to project (hours per week).
Student investigator details	• Identifying and contact details.
	• Time commitment to project (hours per week).
	• Relationship of project to PhD.
Past, current & requested grant funding for all chief investigators (add to list of grants as required)	PAST (awarded past 3 years not including current year):
	• Year & title of grant.
	• Granting body.
	• Administering institution.
	• Investigators.
	• Funding awarded.
	• Brief report (2000 characters max).

(Continued)

APPLICATION

	CURRENT FUNDING (awarded current year):
	• Details as for past funding.
	PENDING FUNDING (applications submitted):
	• Details as for past funding but with requested amount minus a report.
Budget	• Salaries (description, priority, amount requested).
	• Direct research costs (description, priority, amount requested).
	• Staff travel (description, priority, amount requested).
	• Equipment (description, priority, amount requested).
	• Total amount requested.
	• Budget justification (2000 characters max).
	• Funding agency to which a further application for an external grant will be submitted after this project.
	NOTE:
	The importance of each item must be indicated with a priority ranking.
	Salaries should follow relevant university staff classification with appropriate oncosts applied.
	Teaching relief for researchers will not be funded.
Ethics	Committee to which an ethics application has been or will be submitted.
Certification	• Signature of first chief investigator.
	• Signature of the School Dean or delegate.
Research description (max 4 pages)	Project description under the following headings:
	• Aims and significance.
	• Background and research plan.
	• Timetable.
	• References (outside the 4 page limit).
	Font to be no less than 11 point Arial or 12 point Times New Roman and with 2cm page margins all round.

Source: Drawn from the template of the Faculty of Medicine, Nursing and Health Sciences, reproduced with permission from Flinders University of South Australia.

While the application for a small grant, such as the one described above, will take some time, the limit on the information required related to the applicants is for the past 3 years and with a maximum of four pages to describe the project. The length of the application in the case of the example above will be a few pages in excess of 13, depending on how many investigators are added to the team. Attention is paid, in this application, to the potential of the project to lead to a further grant application from an external funding organization.

In Appendix D, at the end of this book, we have provided a second example of a form filler for a large grant. This is from the Emerging Investigator Awards of the Health Research Board of Ireland that is managed through a Grant E-Management System called GEMS. This proposal requires much more detailed information, particularly about the lead investigator, and when completed would run into more than 100 pages. The guidelines accompanying the grant application run to 44 pages. The amount of detail sought is in line with the purpose of the large grant, which is to support the development of talented researchers in academic or research institutions, who are at a critical stage in establishing themselves as independent and self-directed investigators. Beyond the funding to provide support to the researcher, the purpose of the funding is to build collaborative expertise in health services research, hence an application from a researcher to solve a clinical or a biomedical problem would not be applicable to this scheme. Note also the amount of detail needed about the members of the research team and the required description about the collaborative approach that the team will take.

The application for a large grant can be a time-consuming undertaking that requires the gathering of a great deal of information, and that needs to be written up in a detailed way as specified in the template. Care must be taken to ensure that there is not too much repetition of content in parts where there seems to be overlap, for example, such as in the contributions described by individual team members (Appendix D, sections 6 and 7), and the description of the overall team-based approach (section 9). Considerable detail is also requested from co-applicants and official collaborators that requires some effort from them, such as deciding upon and listing relevant publications or the completion of a collaboration agreement. All of these tasks will take time and coordination of effort, and may require some chasing up of research team members to provide the information needed. It is our experience that it is the necessary information from the research team members and obtaining their signatures that can take longer than the writing up of the research plan.

STRATEGIC BUDGETING

One of the areas of grant writing over which applicants are often concerned, and need to seek assistance with, is completing the budget. This is not surprising, as the main reason for writing the application is to seek funds to finance the project. The applicant needs to make sure that the budget items have been adequately costed, particularly to account for any cost rises in the future years over which the project will run and to account for any staff salary or office oncosts.

We have labelled this section 'strategic budgeting' to impress on you that there is a strategy in putting together a budget. The first reason for strategising your budget is that, even if you are successful with your application, you may not be awarded the budget that you asked for. It is our experience that funding agencies generally have less money available than is being sought in worthwhile applications. The funding agency may then cut a percentage off the budget of those highly worthwhile applications on the assumption that applicants can find additional resources elsewhere so that more funds can be awarded to other projects. You will have seen that in the small grant template (Table 7.1) applicants are asked to prioritize budget items so that lower priority items can be removed from the requested budget if a smaller amount is to be awarded. The strategy then is to ask for what is needed, or even a little more, but being prepared to cut the budget in those places where some alternative resourcing arrangement can occur. For instance, travel costs and living expenses in the field can often be reduced, and in-house office expenses such as photocopying can sometimes be absorbed by the host institution. The items that often cannot be cut are research staff salaries, as staff are generally the main resource to conduct the project.

Two areas in the budget that you should seek assistance with are staff salary scales as well as the oncosts and institutional overheads. The cost of employing staff includes the actual salary that would be paid to an individual. The correct classification needs to be determined for the role, skills and qualifications of the staff members you are seeking. Salaries increase because of inflationary moves and also because of progression through salary increments, so forward projections need to be made over the years that the staff will be employed. Second, the oncosts associated with staff employment need to be included, and these will vary for different organizations in different locations, but they need to include the costs of staff leave entitlements, superannuation, workers' compensation insurance, and so on. Also the actual recruitment costs, such as job advertising and travel costs to job interviews, may need to be paid for by the grant. Your organization should be able to calculate these oncosts for you.

One area that may be considered favourably by a funding agency is the inclusion of a PhD scholarship in the application. This shows the funder that you have a focus on building future research capacity. Also, if there is a clear role for a PhD candidate in the research plan this can be a relatively inexpensive way of resourcing some of the research effort.

You will see in the large grant proposal in Appendix D that the application requires the completion of a Gantt Chart. We have always found a Gantt Chart to be helpful in working out what resources will be needed for a project and over what time period these need to be funded. A Gantt Chart lists the main activities of a project down the left column with the time periods of the project at each subsequent column. In the case of Liang's project the time periods are broken up in months (see Table 7.2).

 ACTIVITY 7.2   COMPLETING A GANTT CHART AND A BUDGET

The completion of a Gantt Chart and a budget enable a researcher to determine the resources that will be needed for a project and how much funding to ask for in the grant application. Below are the examples from Liang's proposal. Read this section and reflect on how Liang has constructed his Gantt Chart and budget, particularly his rationale for deciding what resources will be needed.

LIANG'S GANTT CHART

By constructing a Gantt Chart Liang is able to get a good idea of what some of his main expenses, such as staffing and travel, will be. For instance he can now see over

Table 7.2 Gantt Chart: Liang's study on collaborative chronic disease care planning in General Practice

TASK	TIME (months)																							
	1	2	3	4	5	6	7	8	9	10	11	12	13	14	15	16	17	18	19	20	21	22	23	24
Project Advisory Committee	■					■					■							■					■	
Recruit & employ		■																						
...Research Fellow (FT)			■	■	■	■	■	■	■	■	■	■	■	■	■	■	■	■	■	■	■	■	■	■
...Research Fellow (0.5)			■	■	■	■	■	■																■
...Research Assistant (site 1)			■	■	■	■	■	■	■	■	■	■	■	■	■	■	■	■	■	■	■	■	■	■
...Research Assistants (site 2–4)				■	■	■	■	■	■	■	■	■	■	■	■	■	■	■						
Ethics application	■	■	■																					
Develop training materials and measurement tools		■	■	■																				
Recruit General Practices				■	■																			
Conduct training (intervention practices)						■																		
Baseline data collection								■	■															
Follow-up data collection (3 & 6 months)													■	■	■	■	■	■						
Data analysis																			■	■	■			
Conduct training (control practices)																				■				
Reporting																						■	■	■

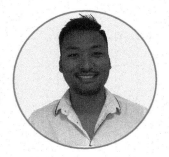

what period he will need to employ staff and when specific expenses such as training and travel costs will be incurred. These will be important considerations, should his grant be awarded in stages, so that he can ensure that there are funds available when accounts are to be paid. Liang was able to show this Gantt Chart to the Senior Administration Officer in his department, in order to gain asssistance to calculate the budget for his proposal.

OUR COMMENTS ON LIANG'S TIMELINE

(THIS INFORMATION WOULD NOT BE INCLUDED IN THE GRANT APPLICATION)

The time taken to recruit appropriate staff can slow the commencement of a project. This includes the time required to prepare position descriptions, seek approval for employment, determine the availability of office space; the time taken to advertise, receive applications, short list and conduct interviews; and the time taken for successful applicants to commence work. This process can easily take up to two months. In Liang's case he already has a senior research fellow and a research assistant in mind who are both interested in the positions, and he has already sought approval to employ these staff on short-term contracts until the longer-term employment processes are completed.

Two months have been allocated for ethics approval. If there are complications with ethics that require a resubmission of the ethics application this approval may take longer. Liang will not be able to commence recruiting General Practices until ethical approval is obtained.

LIANG'S BUDGET

Liang's budget is shown in Table 7.3 below. Note how he has prioritized each budget item on the assumption that, even if successful, he may not get all the funding that he is asking for. For instance he has prioritized the data manager and data analyst items at 3 because he considers that these roles could be added to the duties of the main research fellow and research assistant. He has asked for the level of resources that he would ideally like, knowing that he may have to compromise on this.

Priority

1 = The project will not proceed if not funded at requested level.

2 = Funding is important for the research to proceed in a timely manner as planned.

3 = Funding is important but some adjustment might be possible.

Table 7.3   Budget: Liang's study on collaborative chronic disease care planning in General Practice

STAFF	year 1	year 2	item total	TOTAL	priority
Senior Research Fellow F/T	97,500	105,062	202,562		1
Senior Research Fellow (0.5) @ 6 months	24,375		24,375		3
Research Assistant site 1 (FT) @ 23 months	59,584	35,311	94,895		1
Research Assistants site 2–4 (0.2) @ 14 months	26,016	19,512	45,528		2
Data Manager	5,000	5,000	10,000		3
Data Analyst		10,000	10,000		3
SUBTOTAL STAFF				387,360	
EQUIPMENT					
Laptops @ 6	12,000		12,000		1
SUBTOTAL EQUIPMENT				12,000	
TRAINING					
Training materials	900	900	1800		1
Nurse salary during training	2,370	2,370	4,740		1
TRAINING					
Trainer and participant travel	2,100	2,100	4,200		1
Venue hire & catering	1,000	1,000	2,000		1
SUBTOTAL TRAINING				12,740	
TRAVEL					
Senior Research Fellow to sites	6,000	3,000	9,000		3
Project team meetings	3,000	3,000	6,000		3
Project advisory committee meetings	3,000	2,000	5,000		3
SUBTOTAL TRAVEL				20,000	
PROJECT MANAGEMENT					
Honorarium for 1 Lead GP per Practice	27,000		27,000		2
Consultant to develop Practice business case		7,500	7,500		3
Departmental office costs	25,000	25,000	50,000		3
SUBTOTAL PROJECT MANAGEMENT				84,500	
TOTAL				**516,600**	

JUSTIFICATION OF BUDGET
(INCLUDED IN THE GRANT
APPLICATION)

Staff

- A full-time senior research fellow is required over the 2 year period to conduct the project under the supervision of the chief investigator. This person will be responsible for day to day project management, supervision of the research staff and the organization of the data collection, analysis and reporting. Funding has been costed at the bottom of University Senior Research Fellow salary scale with 30% salary oncosts. For the second year $4000 pa salary increment has been applied along with 2.5% allowance for inflation.
- A second half-time senior research fellow has been included for six months to conduct the training and assist with establishment of the project in the recruited General Practices.
- A full-time research assistant is required over the 23-month period to assist with all aspects of the project including ethics approval, General Practice recruitment, training, the specific data collection from General Practices located at site one, and data analysis and reporting. Funding has been costed at the bottom of University Research Assistant salary scale with the loading applied as per the senior research fellow.
- Three research assistants at one day per week are required over 14 months to conduct the rolling recruitment of patients and collect data from General Practices located at sites two to four.
- A data manager has been nominally costed at $5000 per year. Such a manager is required to ensure the safe and accurate management of data from across 18 General Practices across four sites covering metropolitan and rural locations. The security of data obtained from General Practices is an important consideration that requires careful management.
- A data analyst has been nominally costed at $10,000 for the second year to conduct the statistical work required.

Equipment

Six laptops costed at $2000 each are needed for each of the research staff.

Training

- The cost of developing and printing the training materials has been estimated at $100 per participant with 18 nurses to be trained.
- The nurses' salaries will be covered for the one day training programme costed at $4740.
- Reimbursement for cost of nurses to travel to training has been costed at $100 per nurse and with $600 allocated for the trainer travel costs per training day (4 days).
- Venue hire and catering have been estimated at $500 per training day (4 days).

Travel

- Provision has been made for the senior research fellow to travel to the three external sites, twice in the first year and once in the second year, to establish the project in each site and then for follow-up supervision. Each site visit has been costed at $1000 for travel, accommodation and meals per visit.
- Funding has been allocated for the travel of the staff working at the external site to research team meetings to be held at the research base once per year. Funding has also been nominally estimated for two external members of the project advisory committee to attend the five meetings costed at $500 per member per meeting.

Project management

- General Practices are private businesses reliant on the billing of patients to generate revenue and so time away from seeing patients is lost income. Hence, the time taken by GPs to consider this project and to take part in project discussions is to be nominally funded at an honorarium of $1500 per GP for the lead GPs in each of the 18 Practices.
- The successful adoption of the care coordination model requires that a business case be developed so that Practices can see how they are able to generate sufficient revenue from this new form of service delivery. If the findings show clinical benefit we will contract a business manager to develop a business case, costed at $1500 per day for five days.
- Departmental office costs and university overheads have been costed at approximately 10% of the budget which is below the commercial rate.

OUR COMMENTS ON LIANG'S BUDGET

(THIS INFORMATION WOULD NOT BE INCLUDED IN THE GRANT APPLICATION)

Liang has prioritized the second 0.5 senior research fellow at level three because he knows that the first senior research fellow would be able to conduct the training if needed. While he considers this second 0.5 senior research fellow as desirable, in order to spread the workload at the busy start-up stage, Liang is prepared to cut this position from the project.

The three research assistants for sites two to four have been prioritized at level two because without a staff member per site patient recruitment and data collection will be slower. Liang is prepared to cut one of the positions if needed as he has calculated that along with the other full-time research assistant, he could get by with two additional research assistants rather than three.

Liang considers that a data manager, the data analyst, and the business case consultant would increase the capacity for the smooth running of the project and promote the sustainability of the model after the study is completed. These are the three items that he would cut from the budget if necessary as he knows that the functions that would be performed by these staff could be picked up by the full-time senior research fellow, research assistant, and himself. However, if this were to occur then the workload on these staff would increase and so diminish their capacity to fulfil other duties, such as maintaining communication with participating General Practices and in the drafting of publications.

Travel and departmental office costs have all been prioritized at level three as Liang knows that these items can be altered. The amount of travel can be adjusted, as other technologies such as video conferencing could be used in place of face-to-face meetings. While the departmental overheads have been costed conservatively at around 10% of the overall budget (15% or more is not unusual), Liang knows that some granting agencies will not fund these overheads. While not the case with this scheme, Liang has taken a middle course in asking for some of the budget to cover these overheads, but without seeming to ask for too much. He has cleared this with his Departmental Head who has also agreed not to apply the overhead if the grant agency refuses to fund this item. When calculating provision for university (organizational) overheads you should clear this with the relevant person in authority in writing. This ensures that you have allocated sufficient funds from your budget for this item.

You will note that Liang has estimated the costs for some items, rather than detail actual known costs. Some grant applicants will be more specific and base the budget on quoted actual costs. We recommend that actual costs be included for major items like salaries, as any miscalculation on these items can lead to serious shortfalls. It has been our experience that informed estimates for items like computers, travel, and catering are sufficient. Experience has shown us that while actual expenditures generally follow the budget estimates broadly, as a project proceeds this will not be exact, with some budget lines going over and others going under. Hence, we have found that having the permission to move funding between lines on the budget is desirable.

Our final comment on budgeting is that you should use the formula function on a spreadsheet to calculate the budget. Manually working out a budget increases the chances that you will make a calculation error, particularly if you make progressive alterations to specific items that require a recalculation of subtotal and totals each time.

 ACTIVITY 7.3   YOUR GANTT CHART AND BUDGET

Having read how Liang has constructed a Gantt Chart and budget, and how he has made strategic decisions about these, now construct a Gantt Chart and budget for your project. If your project is small, the detail and skills required to construct these will be less than that required for a large grant.

APPENDICES, LETTERS OF SUPPORT

Having put together your funding proposal you can now add attachments to the application to provide evidence of the support that you have secured that will enable you to conduct the project. Different funding templates will specify what attachments are required and commonly these can include the curriculum vitae of the chief investigators and also letters (on institutional letterhead) from the administrating and participating organizations that describe how they will support and be involved in the project.

COMMITTEE PROCESSES

WHICH PANEL FOR PEER REVIEW

If the funding scheme that you are applying to is a small one, there may be no decision about which subcommittee will review your application. There may be only one committee. For large grant schemes that receive many applications, subcommittees or panels will often be convened in order to review applications that fall within different areas, so that a different subcommittee will review applications for different scientific disciplines or different topic areas. Such schemes will often provide applicants with the opportunity to identify which subcommittee they consider is most appropriate to review their application. This can be stated on the application template or by the choice of keywords or field of research classification codes that are published by funding organizations. It is important to target an application to the most appropriate subcommittee to ensure that committee members and peer reviewers are those with the methodological and topic expertise relevant to your application. In this way, your application is most likely to receive the best review because the committee members and peer reviewers will then have the background to understand your proposed topic and research methods. Even if well targeted, it is not always the case that a subcommittee will have members who are informed and familiar with all of the topics and methodologies of the applications sent to them.

As an illustration, the indicative panels for the 2017 round of project grants for the Australian National Health and Medical Research Council (undated) are listed below:

- Clinical Trials + Cohort Studies.
- Dentistry + Surgery + Medical Technologies + Primary Care + Nutrition + Nursing and Midwifery.
- Health Services + Health Promotion + Ageing + Allied Health.
- Neuroscience (incl Vision Science & Audiology) + Dementia.
- Endocrinology + Diabetes + Gastroenterology + Musculoskeletal + Obesity.
- Genetics + Molecular Biology + Bioinformatics & Computational Biology.
- Immunology + Inflammation + Rheumatology.

- Microbiology + Virology.
- Mental Health + Psychology + Psychiatry.
- Pharmacology + Respiratory Medicine + Sleep Disorders.
- Biochemistry + Cell Biology + Regenerative Medicine + Developmental Biology.
- Cardiovascular Disease + Nephrology (incl Haematology).
- Cancer Biology + Oncology (incl Haematological Tumours).
- Reproductive Medicine + Obstetrics & Gynaecology + Paediatrics.
- Epidemiology + Population Health.
- Indigenous Health.

You can see that some panels cover a wide topic range (like dentistry to nursing) while others are more specific (like immunology to rheumatology). This classification of some panels into highly specialised areas and others into more generalist areas does mean that researchers should carefully consider how to write their application so that it will be sent to the panel with the skills to provide the best review. Those applications that propose novel scientific methodologies can face scepticism from panel members not familiar with the value and rigour conventions of new methodologies.

REJOINDERS

Having submitted your application, you have the time to wait until you receive information back from the funding organization. For smaller grants, the time period may only be a few months and the first notification from the organization may be their decision about whether your application has been successful or not. For larger grants, the waiting time could be six months or more and the first notification sent to you may be the reports of the peer reviewers that have not yet been considered by the review subcommittee. These peer review reports are provided to give you the opportunity to respond to the reviewers' critique. The response is often called a rejoinder and this will be added to the material that will be used by the subcommittee to make a decision about your application. It is important to consider the critique carefully and to use this constructively, either to diplomatically disagree with certain critique if you can do this, or to use the critique to improve elements of the study design, so long as this keeps the study within the scope of what has been proposed.

TOP TIP

Two golden rules of rejoinders:

1. Always respond even if the critique is so bad that it seems pointless. You are showing yourself to the scientific community and, as reputations are built over time, how you respond now may influence how panellists will continue to view you later.

2. Never come across as being defensive or angry in a rejoinder. Even if a peer reviewer seems not to have understood your application, use this as an opportunity to re-explain (briefly) the aspect of your application that has been critiqued. There is a good chance that the subcommittee members may also see your application in the same way as the peer reviewer, and these committee members will not consider favourably a defensive or angry rejoinder from you.

CONCLUSION

This final chapter has taken you through Step Seven, the final step in writing a research proposal, that is, in submitting an application for funding. By now you will have realised that writing a research proposal can be a demanding activity that involves many steps that need to be followed in a logical sequence in order to arrive at the end point – that end point being a completed application ready for submission. Like any large task, if approached in a systematic and planned way and with adequate time and assistance, what may have seemed daunting at the start can be achieved. Even if a proposal is not approved at the first submission, there is the reward in having completed a good proposal that can be used as the basis for refinement and resubmission or alternatively submitted to another funding organization.

We hope that you have found this step-by-step guide helpful and enjoyed working through the stages of writing up your own proposal. We wish you well in your research endeavours and in your pursuit of knowledge.

REVISION

Below you will find five statements related to the content of this chapter. Indicate whether you believe each statement to be true or false. The answers are given on p. 150.

1. It is a good idea to submit lots of grant applications on the probability that at least one will succeed.

   T/F

2. A Gantt Chart enables the researcher to determine what resources will be needed and over what time period these will be needed.

   T/F

3. It is better to include some non-critical items in your budget on the assumption that, if approved, you will not be awarded the funding amount that you asked for.

   T/F

4. If you target your application carefully, then the members of review committees will always come from the discipline background that is familiar with your topic and methodology.

   T/F

5. When completing a rejoinder it is best to reply forcefully and defend your stance.

   T/F

REFERENCES

Flinders University (undated) Grants Bulletin. (www.flinders.edu.au/research/researcher-support/grants-contracts/search/grants-bulletin.cfm). [last accessed 5 September 2017]

National Health and Medical Research Council (undated) Advice to applicants on choosing their peer review area. (www.nhmrc.gov.au/_files_nhmrc/file/grants/apply/projects/attachment_1_advice_to_applicants_on_choosing_their_peer_review_area_in_2017_v0-03.pdf). [last accessed 29 August 2017]

ANSWERS TO ACTIVITIES

REVISION

1. = F
2. = T
3. = T
4. = F
5. = F

You can find Appendix D on sections in a template for a large grant at the end of this book.

APPENDICES

APPENDIX A: CRITICAL REVIEW GUIDELINES FOR QUALITATIVE STUDIES

Title and abstract

a. Is the title of the research paper concise, clear and congruent with the text?
b. Are the aims and/or objectives stated? What are they?
c. Does the abstract contain sufficient information about the stages of the research process (e.g. aims, research, approach, participants, data collection, data analysis, findings)?

Identifying the phenomenon/phenomena of interest

a. Is the phenomenon focused on human experience within a natural setting?
b. Is the phenomenon relevant to nursing, midwifery and/or health?

Structuring the study

a. Is it clear that the selected participants have experience of the phenomenon of interest?
b. How is published literature used in the study?
c. Does the question identify the context (participant/group/place) of the method to be followed?
d. Is the theoretical framework clearly stated?
e. Does the theoretical framework fit the research question?
f. Is the method of data collection and analysis clearly specified?
g. Does the qualitative method of data collection chosen fit the research question (e.g. grounded theory, ethnography)?
h. Are the limitations of the study stated?

Research question and design

a. Was the research question determined by the need for the study? How was this determination made?
b. Are the data collection strategies appropriate for the research question?
c. Do the data collection strategies reflect the purpose and theoretical framework of the study (e.g. in-depth interviewing, focus groups)?
d. Can the data analysis strategy be identified and logically followed?

Participants

a. How were the participants and setting selected (e.g. sampling strategies)?
b. How was confidentiality of the participants assured?
c. How was the anonymity of participants assured?
d. What ethical issues were identified in the study?
e. How were the ethical issues addressed?

Data analysis

a. How were the data analysed?
b. Is the analysis technique congruent with the research question?
c. Is there evidence that the researcher's interpretation captured the participant's meaning?
d. Did the researcher say how the criteria for judging the scientific rigour of the study were maintained in terms of credibility, auditability, fittingness and confirmability?

Describing the findings

a. Does the researcher demonstrate to the reader the method (e.g. audit trial) by which the data were analysed?
b. Does the researcher indicate how the findings are related to theory?
c. Is there a link between the findings to existing theory or literature, or is a new theory generated?

Researcher's perspective

a. Are the biases of the researcher reported (e.g. researcher/participant expectations, researcher bias and power imbalance)?
b. Are the limitations of the study acknowledged?
c. Are recommendations suggested for further research?
d. Are implications for health care mentioned?

Source: Schneider et al., (2016) *Nursing and Midwifery Research: methods and appraisal for evidence-based practice* 5th edn. Australia: Elsevier. Reproduced with permission.

APPENDIX B: CRITICAL REVIEW GUIDELINES FOR QUANTITATIVE STUDIES

Title and abstract

a. Is the title of the research paper congruent with the text?
b. Are the aims and/or objectives stated? What are they?
c. Does the abstract contain sufficient information about the stages of the research process (e.g. aims, hypothesis, research approach, sample, instruments and findings)?

Structuring the study

a. Is the motivation for the study demonstrated through the literature review?
b. Is the literature cited current, relevant and comprehensive? Are the references recent?
c. Are the stated limitations and gaps in the reviewed literature appropriate and convincing?
d. How was the investigation carried out?
e. Is the hypothesis stated?
f. Which hypothesis is stated: the scientific hypothesis or the null hypothesis?
g. Does the hypothesis indicate that the researcher is interested in testing for differences between groups or in testing relationships?

The sample

a. Is the sample described?
b. Is the sample size large enough to prevent an extreme score from affecting the summary statistics used?
c. How was the sample size determined?
d. Is the sample size appropriate for the analyses used?

Data collection

a. How were the data collected (questionnaires or other data collection tools)?
b. Who collected the data?
c. Are the data adequately described?
d. What is the origin of the measurement instruments?
e. Are the instruments adequately described?
f. How were the data collection instruments validated?

g. How was the reliability of the measurement instruments assessed?
h. Were ethical issues discussed?

Data analysis

a. Are descriptive or inferential statistics reported?
b. What tests were used to analyse the data: parametric or non-parametric?
c. Were the descriptive statistics/inferential statistics appropriate to the level of measurement for each variable?
d. Were the appropriate tests used to analyse the data?
e. What is the level of measurement chosen for the independent and dependent variables?
f. Were the statistics appropriate for the research question and design?
g. Are there appropriate summary statistics for each major variable?
h. Were the statistics primarily descriptive, correlational or inferential?
i. Identify the outcome of each statistical analysis
j. Explain the meaning of each outcome

Findings

a. Were the findings expected? Which findings were not expected?
b. Is there enough information present to judge the results?
c. Are the results clearly and completely stated?
d. Describe the researcher's report of the findings
e. Identify any limitations or gaps in the study
f. Were suggestions for further research made?
g. Did the researcher mention the implications of the study for health care?
h. Was there sufficient information in the report to permit replication of the study?

Source: Schneider et al., (2016) *Nursing and Midwifery Research: methods and appraisal for evidence-based practice* 5th edn. Australia: Elsevier. Reproduced with permission.

APPENDIX C (1)

NATASHA'S INFORMATION SHEET AND CONSENT FORM

INFORMATION SHEET

This is an example of an information sheet to be printed on the letterhead of the agency/hospital/university at which you are enrolled/employed.

Dear _____

I am currently studying for my *(name of degree)* at *(name of university)*. My dissertation is by research. The title of my research project is:

'Women's experiences of anxiety and fear in the first trimester of pregnancy: a qualitative study.'

Researcher: (student's name, department in which enrolled, university, suburb, state and postcode).

_____

_____

Telephone number/mobile: _____

Email: _____

Address: _____

My supervisors are: Dr M. Green (Hospital X) and Dr C. Maunders (University X).

I would like to invite you to consider participating in my research project. The purpose of this qualitative study is to discover your personal experiences of feelings of anxiety and fear in the first trimester of pregnancy. I am asking you to share your unique experiences and interpretation of your feelings in an audio-recorded interview in your home. I would also like you to complete two questionnaires at the interview.

Your participation in this study and any information you provide will be kept confidential. Your name will be replaced with a pseudonym (a number or fictitious name). All your information will be kept in a locked place. My supervisors will have access to your information but not your name or any of your details.

I do not anticipate any risks (emotional or physical discomfort) to you in this study.

Since little is known about how women experience anxiety and fear during the first trimester of pregnancy, I hope that whatever we learn from this research study will benefit women and do much to ensure a happy, comfortable and safe pregnancy and delivery.

If you agree to participate, you will be asked to attend (a) one audio-recorded interview lasting about 1 – 1½ hours conducted in your home before the 14th week of pregnancy, and (b) to complete a questionnaire about how you cope, that is, your coping strategies. The interview will be conducted at a mutually convenient time.

Please understand that you are free to withdraw from participation in the research study at any time and ask that all your audio-recorded and written records be returned to you or destroyed and not used in any way, provided that your request be made within 4 weeks of the completion of the interview.

You may ask for a copy of this document for your own records. You may also request information about the findings of the study.

Any complaint regarding the nature or conduct of this research may be directed to:

Ethics Liaison Officer, Human Research Ethics Committee *(name of university/agency, suburb, state, postcode)*

_____

_____

Telephone: _____ Date: _____

Thank you for taking time to read this information sheet.

Yours sincerely,

(Researcher's name)

APPENDIX C (2)

CONSENT FORM

This is an example of a consent form to be printed on the letterhead of the agency/hospital/university at which you are enrolled/employed.

Title of Project: 'Women's experiences of anxiety and fear in the first trimester of pregnancy: a qualitative study.'

Name of researcher and agency address: _____

_____

I, *(name of participant) (please print)* have read and understood all of the information on the information sheet and any questions that I have asked have been answered to my satisfaction.

I agree to take part in this research study on the understanding that:

- I can withdraw from the study at any stage
- I agree to the one interview, in my home, being taped
- I complete two questionnaires at the time of my interview
- I agree to the use of any material which does not identify me in any way

I understand that I am free to withdraw from participation in this research study at any time after my interview and ask that my audio-recorded and written records be returned to me or destroyed and not used in any way, provided that the request for destruction or return of records be made within 4 weeks of the completion of the interview.

Should I wish to discuss my participation with someone not directly involved in the research project, particularly in respect to matters concerning policies, information about the conduct of the study, or my rights as a participant, or I wish to make a confidential complaint, I may contact:

Ethics Liaison Officer, Human Research Ethics Committee, *(name of university/agency, suburb, state, postcode)*

_____

_____

Telephone: _____

Name of Participant: _____ **Researcher:**_____

Date:_____ Signature:_____ Date:_____ Signature:_____

APPENDIX D: SECTIONS IN A TEMPLATE FOR A LARGE GRANT

Scheme name	Emerging Investigator Awards for Health
	Health Research Board, Ireland
Purpose	• Support and nurture talented individuals at a critical career stage establishing themselves as independent and self-directed researchers.
	• Establish a cadre of collaborative experts who can generate new knowledge in health research … towards improving health care systems, policies or practice.
Eligibility	• Health-related researchers or professionals with at least 4 years since the award of a PhD;
	• Who can demonstrate five significant contributions to scientific knowledge with at least four references per contribution;
	• Who has at least 3 years post-doctoral (or related) professional experience;
	• Who has NOT been the lead investigator on a grant from the HRB that is greater than 100,000 euro;
	• Who does NOT have an established team as an independent principal investigator;
	• Who does not hold a faculty position with an end date more than 2 years from the submission due date of the application.
Funding items covered	• Salary of the lead applicant and research personnel
	• Research-related costs of the first project
	• Institutional overheads (30% for laboratory and 25% for desk based research)
	• Maximum 800,000 euros over 4 years
Assessment criteria	50% – expertise of the lead applicant
	30% – the research project
	20% – support and environment

APPLICATION

Summary (1 page)	Title, lead applicant, mentor, co-applicants, host institution, duration (months), budget total, abstract

1. Project details

Project title	Maximum 200 characters
Project duration	Number of months
Grant start date	
Project lay summary	Maximum 300 words: include objectives, design, expected outcomes and anticipated benefit in a plain English language summary.
Project abstract	Maximum 300 words: succinct stand-alone summary.
Keywords	

(Continued)

APPLICATION

2. Lead applicant

Personal details	Name, contact details, institution, profession and membership of professional bodies
Education	Dates, degree, institution, country, subject
Employment	Dates, job title, employer
Funding record	Dates, duration, amount, title, funding body, reference number, role
Personal declaration	Maximum 600 words: why you are suited to the role as an emerging investigator and your potential as an independent researcher. Reference up to four of your research outputs most relevant to this application.
Research contributions (up to 5)	Contributions to scientific knowledge. Describe up to five of your most significant intellectual contributions to scientific knowledge. For each contribution describe the following:

- The background to the idea and the scientific question
- The main findings
- The influence/impact of the findings
- Your role in the research
- Up to four outputs from the research

3. Research project description

Research question	Maximum 200 words
Background	Maximum 1000 words: background to the research proposal including the size and nature of the issue.
Overall aim	Maximum 100 words
Objectives	For each objective, state the deliverables in bullet point format. Include a Gantt Chart with objectives and deliverables against timelines.
Research design and methodological approach	Maximum 4000 words: summarize the proposed research plan, with description of individual streams of work and how they integrate to form a coherent proposal.
Pathway to actionable knowledge	Maximum 600 words: describe how the research will be applied towards improving the health care system, policies or practices.
Dissemination and knowledge exchange plan	Maximum 600 words: how the outputs will be disseminated and made openly accessible.
Project management	Maximum 600 words: how the project will be managed.
Public involvement in the research	Maximum 600 words: how the public has been involved in the preparation and/or design of this application and proposed future involvement.
Data management and sharing plan	The data management during and after the project
References	Maximum 30
Gender issues in the research	Maximum 500 words
Potential risks and ethical concerns	Maximum 400 words
Compliance with data protection regulations	Maximum 300 words

4. Infrastructure and support

Infrastructure and support	Maximum 400 words: the facilities, expertise and other support at the host institution.

5. Research team: mentor

Mentor	Name and contact details
Education	Dates, degree, institution, country, subject
Employment	Dates, job title, employer
Grants	Dates, duration, amount, title, funding body, reference number, role
Evidence of leadership and collaborative role	Maximum 400 words: reference up to four research outputs relevant to this expertise/role.
Evidence of expertise translated into health care practice, policy or service delivery	Maximum 400 words: reference up to four research outputs relevant to this expertise/role.
Evidence of capacity building, mentoring and coaching	Maximum 400 words: reference up to four research outputs relevant to this expertise/role.

6. Research team: co-applicants (add section for each applicant)

Personal details	Name, contact details, institution, profession and membership of professional bodies
Education	Dates, degree, institution, country, subject
Employment	Dates, job title, employer
Funding record	Dates, duration, amount, title, funding body, reference number, role.
Personal declaration	Maximum 400 words: why you are suited to the role as a co-applicant for this proposal. Reference up to four of your research outputs most relevant to this application.
Research contributions (up to five)	Contributions to scientific knowledge. Describe up to five of your most significant intellectual contributions to scientific knowledge. For each contribution (350 words) describe the following: • The background to the idea and the scientific question • The main findings • The influence/impact of the findings • Your role in the research • Up to four outputs from the research

7. Research team: official collaborators (add section for each collaborator)

Personal details	Name, institution, position, academic and professional qualifications, previous positions held over past 5 years.
Collaborator's role	
Publications	Maximum 200 words: list up to five of the collaborator's publications relevant to this application.
Grants	Maximum 200 words: list past and current grants in which the collaborator was a lead or co-applicant that are relevant to this application.
Agreement	Attach a signed collaborator agreement that describes the objectives of the collaboration (150 words), the collaborator's contribution to the project

(Continued)

APPLICATION

(150 words), how the collaboration will enable the research to proceed (150 words), any conflicts of interest (150 words), restrictions on technology or knowledge transfer or dissemination of results (150 words) and any additional or in-kind income or expenditure to the collaborator arising from the project with justification (200 words).

8. Research team: research personnel

Personnel details	Personnel type, % on the project, role
Justification	Provide justification for the personnel relative to the scale and complexity of the project.
Higher degree/ postgraduate students	Indicate involvement of higher degree/postgraduate students in the project.

9. Collaborative and team-based approach

Team	Maximum 600 words: describe why you have chosen the research team members and the overall complementarity of skills and disciplines.
Mentor arrangements	Maximum 200 words: describe why you have chosen this mentor and how the mentoring arrangements will work.

10. Research and professional development plan

Research and professional development plan	Maximum 500 words: describe the training and professional development activities that you wish to undertake to support your application as an independent researcher.

11. Institutional support to the lead applicant

Institutional support	Provide a letter of support from the host institution indicating the nature of the support and the benefit of the project to the host institution.

12. Project budget

Staff (list for each staff)	Type, classification, basic salary and employer salary on costs with justification (per year)
Running costs	List per item per year with justification
Equipment	List per item per year with justification
Dissemination	List per item per year with justification
Overheads	Add percentage per year

13. Ethical approvals

Ethical approvals	List the ethical approvals that are required.

14. Appendices

Gantt Chart
Collaborator agreements
Institutional letter of support

Source: Template of the Emerging Investigator Awards of the Health Research Board of Ireland. Reproduced with permission.

INDEX

Figures and Tables are indicated by page numbers in bold print.